C·R·E·A·T·I·O·N Health
DISCOVERY

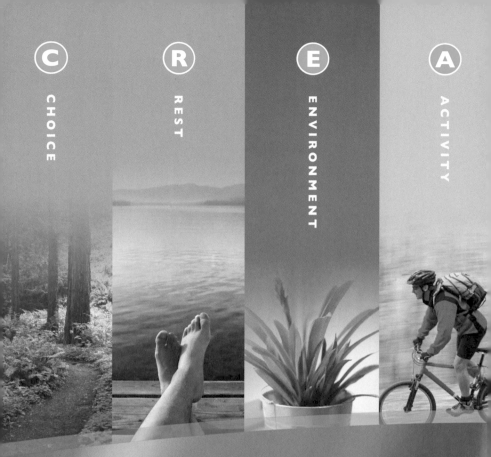

C CHOICE

R REST

E ENVIRONMENT

A ACTIVITY

Des Cummings Jr., PhD

with Monica Reed, MD

and Todd Chobotar

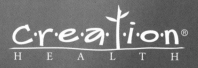

creation®
HEALTH

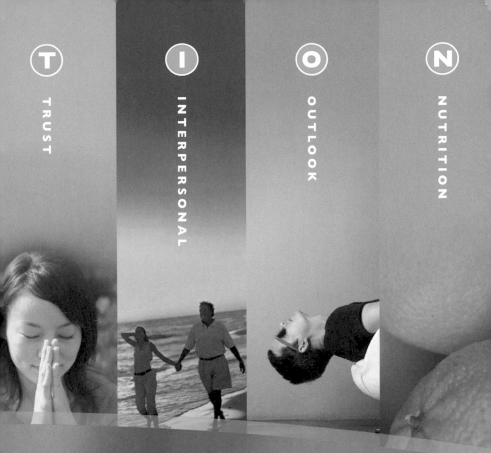

T TRUST

I INTERPERSONAL

O OUTLOOK

N NUTRITION

C·R·E·A·T·I·O·N Health
DISCOVERY

YOUR PATH TO A HEALTHY 100

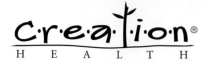

CREATION HEALTH DISCOVERY
Fifth Edition
Copyright © 2005, 2008, 2011, 2014 Des Cummings Jr.
Published by Florida Hospital Publishing
900 Winderley Place, Suite 1600, Maitland, FL 32751

TO EXTEND *the* HEALTH *and* HEALING MINISTRY *of* CHRIST

Editor-in-Chief	Todd Chobotar
Managing Editor	David Biebel, DMin
Promotion	Laurel Prizigley
Production	Lillian Boyd
Copy Editor	Pam Nordberg
Photography	Spencer Freeman
Cover Design	Carter Design
Interior Design	Timothy Brown

PUBLISHER'S NOTE: This book is not intended to replace a one-on-one relationship with a qualified healthcare professional but as a sharing of knowledge and information from the research and experience of the author. You are advised and encouraged to consult with your healthcare professional in all matters relating to your health and the health of your family. The publisher and authors disclaim any liability arising directly or indirectly from the use of this book.

AUTHORS' NOTE: This book contains many case histories and patient stories. In order to preserve the privacy of some of the people involved, we have disguised names, appearances, and aspects of their personal stories so they are not identifiable. Patient stories may also include composite characters.

Unless otherwise noted, all Scripture quotations are from the Holy Bible, New International Version. Copyright © 1973, 1978, 1984, International Bible Society. Used by permission of Zondervan. All rights reserved. Texts credited to NKJV are from the New King James Version. Copyright © 1979, 1982 by Thomas Nelson. Used by permission. All rights reserved. Scripture marked NLT are taken from the Holy Bible, New Living Translation, Copyright © 1996. Used by permission of Tyndale House Publishers, Inc., Wheaton, IL 60189. All translations used by permission.

For volume discounts please contact special sales at:
HealthProducts@FLHosp.org | 407-303-1929

Library of Congress Control Number: 2014932885:
Printed in the United States of America
ISBN-13: 978-0-9839881-8-2
PR 15 14 13 12 11 10 9 8 7 6 5

For other life changing resources visit:
FloridaHospitalPublishing.com
Healthy100Churches.org
CreationHealth.com
Healthy100.org

Contents

What would you say if someone offered you a way to find more energy for your day?

....

What if you could enjoy better daily health?

....

Want a longer life?

....

Would you like to know how to recover more quickly from illness?

....

Do you wish your relationships were strong and peace filled?

....

Do you desire more joy and peace of mind during each day?

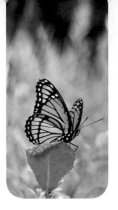

CREATION Health

CHAPTER I

The Original Formula for Feeling Great

THIS COULD BE THE MOST IMPORTANT BOOK YOU will read this year. It will help you experience life at its very best and find new energy and peace. The ideas you find here could turn your whole life upside down—*for the better!*

Now, before you get nervous, let me tell you what this book won't do. It won't demand that you go on a broccoli-only diet, that you run twelve miles each day, or that you start taking ten-minute "power-naps" each hour.

I would love to tell you that the secret of optimum health is eating an ice-cream bar every afternoon, but this book is not about fads or extremes—it's about learning a new way to think about your life.

Sound simple? It is—and it isn't. The concept is simple—eight easy-to-remember steps to a new life. But like everything good, the process calls for commitment, energy, and time. Yet it will bring rewards far beyond anything the stock market has ever offered.

You can have a better life! The best life!

Why should you even want a better life? Why should you go to the effort to incorporate changes to your life when perhaps you're living a pretty good life already?

For many, the goal will simply be to start feeling better every day, to quit getting sick as often, to lose some weight, to sleep better at night, to get the heart rate down, and ratchet the *outlook on life* meter up a few more notches. Great goals, but there's more to all of this than simply making your own day better.

You've got to live longer for the generations behind you.

Whether it's your children or grandchildren, people on this earth need what you can offer—you! If you don't do what you can to live better and live longer, then all of the significant people you love in your life may miss out on years of joy you could have spent encouraging and loving them.

This book isn't just about helping make you into a better you, it's about being around to leave the legacy you want to leave.

THIS IS FOR YOU!

You may be cracking open this book and wondering, *Why do I need another health book? I'm in decent shape. I eat pretty well. I sleep okay. How can this book help me?*

No matter what level of health you may have, the principles in this book can take you even higher. And should you not be happy with your present health, this book can get you feeling and looking great.

And if you are feeling pretty good but could use a little energy boost, *CREATION Health*® will lead you to new ways of increasing your vitality and adding a brighter sparkle to your eye. *CREATION Health* can even add new certainty to a teenager's step. For those entering their fifties or sixties or seventies (or better!), this book offers practical solutions for making every day a better day.

Sound unbelievable?

Read on and you will become a believer because you'll begin to grasp a realistic and doable model of what life ought to be. And none of what you read will have any taste of fad to it. The eight principles described are as old as time and have been tested through the ages.

SUCCESS STORIES OF REAL PEOPLE

CREATION Health isn't a plan filled with esoteric psychotransformational concepts and giant words. It's about proven facts, individual tales of change, improvement, new energy, and peace.

You'll encounter a chaplain who turned his life around through becoming physically active. You'll meet a lawyer who learned to slow down and, in the process, found his family. And you'll read the story of a cancer researcher who got cancer himself and how his network of close relationships helped him recover. Through these stories and more, you'll learn the principles that can change your life as well.

When people decide to alter their lives—when they make personal commitments to make wiser choices, to enjoy adequate rest, to celebrate the best in their environment, and more—amazing things happen.

This book will introduce you to real people who have moved beyond depression, who have lost weight, who have fixed broken relationships, and who can finally wake up without fear. Something big you'll quickly grasp is 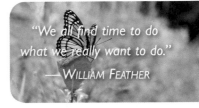 how interconnected life truly is. After all, what good is it to lick cancer if your kids despise you? To lose weight and then put it back on right after the holidays? To walk a brisk five miles but don't know where you are going in this life or the next?

"We all find time to do what we really want to do."
—WILLIAM FEATHER

I will make you a promise about what you'll read. The stories in these pages won't ever be about people who bought into "before and after" quick-fix miracle cures. They are accounts of men and women who decided they wanted to experience complete health—mentally, physically, spiritually, and socially—and who followed the *CREATION Health* principles to get there.

HOW THIS BOOK CAN REENERGIZE YOU

First, I hope to inspire you that there is a better way to live the one life you've been given.

Second, it will demonstrate that you can get there!

And third, it will teach you how to master the eight most powerful principles for improving every part of your life.

You will discover the scientific research behind each of the eight principles—carefully designed studies, performed by major universities and institutes—that point the way to enjoying the best health possible.

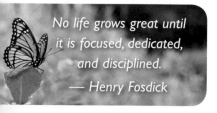

No life grows great until it is focused, dedicated, and disciplined.

— Henry Fosdick

Reliable medical experts will share simple life-improvement tools you can use today.

You will learn the best ways to eat, exercise, and create a balanced healing environment in your life. And you might even be inspired to join others—maybe your own family—in making a commitment to change for the better.

WHERE CREATION HEALTH CAME FROM

The Adventist Health System was founded on the belief that God intended us to enjoy both health and healing. God's model for health is found in the Creation story. In seven magnificent days he fashioned a world in which humans could experience full life and full love. Tragically, this world was shattered, and the majestic garden of life became a jungle of death. But God chose to intervene by coming to earth in person. For thirty-three years he brought a glimpse of the garden to those trapped in the jungle. The greatest part of his time on earth was spent healing the sick.

It is from this example that the Adventist Health System was inspired to build hospitals that we may continue to extend the healing touch of God to a hurting world. What makes these hospitals unique is that we seek to do three things:

1. Treat each person as a child of God;

2. Heal the mind, body, and spirit;

3. Inspire each patient to experience CREATION Health.

We believe you are a special gift from God, and it is our sacred privilege to care for you in sickness and in health. We believe that you can experience optimum healing when we provide the finest diagnostics and therapies to meet your physical needs and compassionate care to calm your emotions and inspire your spirit. This is our mission and our hope for you.

Although the principles of healthy living have been a part of our philosophy for more than 100 years, the CREATION Health lifestyle program came about more recently. A few years ago, one hospital in the Adventist Health System was faced with a unique challenge. The Walt Disney Corporation dreamed of building a new community near Orlando called Celebration. One of Disney's goals for this new community was to create the "healthiest town in America." To accomplish such a big dream, they needed a healthcare partner with a big vision. In stepped Florida Hospital.

Drawing on the Adventist Health System philosophy of "Whole Person Health"—taken from the Creation story—the medical team defined eight principles for CREATION Health. These principles were used to create a new, groundbreaking hospital in the town of Celebration, a hospital that would focus on both health and healing. The CREATION Health principles were used in the hospital's architecture, its medical care, its fitness center, and its customer service. We have found that following the CREATION Health principles does more than change lives—it also transforms the way we do business. For the better!

There's even more to the story of CREATION Health that you can explore on a special Internet web site at *CreationHealth.com*.

HOW CREATION HEALTH WORKS

If you're a bit averse to reading or hearing about how God designed life, this book may be a bit tough to get into. Not that we're going to preach about anything here in these pages. That won't happen. But if you are fairly convinced you aren't a cosmic accident, that perhaps a wise Creator made humans qualitatively different for a reason, and that as a wise Designer he may have left a few "design particulars" that should be followed for the proper care, upkeep, and smooth running of your planet earth suit . . . then this book will have tons of great information for you to consider.

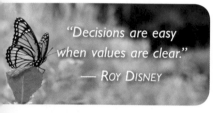

"Decisions are easy when values are clear."
— ROY DISNEY

The truth is, since the dawn of time humans have been blessed with good gifts. At some point in Creation our spectacular planet began brimming with life—flying, swimming, crawling, waddling, growing, blooming life. Many believe that in the center of it all was a garden called Eden, a haven God planted as a gift for his first two children, Adam and Eve. Along with their new garden home, one of the first and finest gifts that was given to them was abundant, full health—physical health, mental health, social health, and spiritual health. By closely examining this "CREATION Health," we learn much about feeling fit and living long and fulfilling lives today. These principles first established for wellness are timeless.

Full health is more than the absence of disease and its symptoms; it is a moment-by-moment realization that God wants each human being on earth—people like you and me whom he loves and cares about—to have the absolute best that this life can offer. Is there any parent who doesn't want the best for their child? No, and so it makes sense that God would want his best for us. Naturally, human choice sometimes makes life messy, so not everything can or will be perfect as it once was. But that doesn't mean we ought not take a hard look at the earliest records of humans found in the Bible to see if there isn't something special that can be gleaned.

That's what the mission team did years ago. After reading and re-reading the Genesis account of Creation, and after spending many hours considering God's plans for health, the team chose to use CREATION Health as an easy-to-remember acronym for full health. The letters of the acronym stand for:

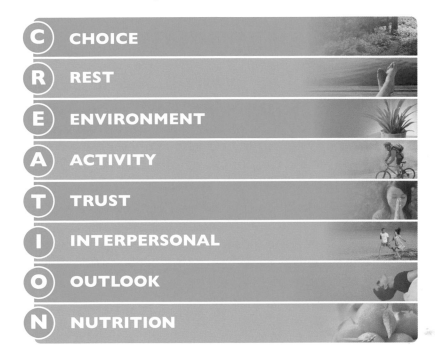

C CHOICE

R REST

E ENVIRONMENT

A ACTIVITY

T TRUST

I INTERPERSONAL

O OUTLOOK

N NUTRITION

In this book I've taken these principles and transformed them into a handful of easy-to-follow steps. We've discovered that embracing the CREATION Health prescription can restore health, happiness, balance, and joy. These eight principles are God's gift to help us experience life as he designed us to live it.

As we unpack the principles in this book, there's something important to keep in mind. Our focus on healthy living doesn't make God love us any more or less. Living a healthy life is not something to boast about or feel proud about; it is only our humble response to his grace and mercy that motivates us to pursue health in order to do the work God has given us to do. For "...the kingdom of God is not eating and drinking, but righteousness and peace and joy in the Holy Spirit" (Romans 14:17, NKJV) and we are saved by grace, through faith… not of works, lest anyone should boast" (see Ephesians 2:8,9). So together, let's pursue health not to be loved, but because we are already loved.

WHAT'S NEXT?

Before you turn to chapter 2 and begin the next step on your CREATION Health journey, let me share one more insight about health and wellness.

All of us want to live without sickness, to have healthy legs, sharp eyes, and quick minds. We want to be healed from everything unhealthy, and we would prefer not having to worry about cancer, accidents, and aging. Desiring to be healthy is good.

But CREATION Health is about wellness, and wellness is more than health or absence of disease. Wellness is being mentally fit, physically robust, spiritually vital, and socially comfortable. It is being able to face accidents, aging, and illness with a positive outlook. Most of all, it is trusting that a loving and kind God has a "better idea" for living and that he is eager to help us experience full life—*as he created us to live it!*

Welcome to CREATION Health, God's prescription for living.

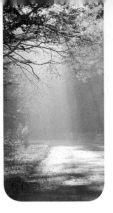

ARE YOU LIVING CREATION HEALTHY?

Take the free CREATION Health quiz online and find out.

DO YOU HAVE 10 MINUTES TO FIND OUT HOW HEALTHY you really are? Go to *www.CREATIONHealth.com*. The CREATION Health self-assessment takes just ten minutes and will help determine the areas where you can focus more attention on your health.

Other helpful things you'll find on the website:

- Read an inspirational devotional to encourage you.

- CREATION Health Conversations: ninety-second videos that make the science of wellness simple and fun

- Daily health tips to keep you on track

- How to download the CREATION Health App to stay on your wellness plan

- Discover new resources for your healthy lifestyle, including books, videos, seminars, music, conferences, and other resources.

WWW.CREATIONHEALTH.COM

Do you sometimes feel other people's choices affect you more than your own?

....

Have you made big decisions in the past but usually wound up with small results?

....

Do you think you have no say-so in your life; that it is predetermined by someone you can't see and don't trust?

....

Are you able to see where your current choices are taking you?

....

Do you believe that you inherited poor health and cannot change?

....

Would you like to start making better, more realistic choices today?

....

The "C" in CREATION Health stands for Choice.

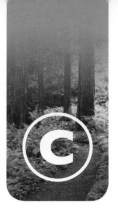

CHOICE

CHAPTER 2

The Secret of Your Success

WE ARE WHAT WE CHOOSE. SOME OF OUR CHOICES are important to daily life but have no moral impact. However, many decisions contain moral challenges, powerful options that could change the direction of life. And most of these choices aren't of the big life-changing variety. They're the "one degree" choices that over time take us far off of our intended goal.

Very few people start their adult life and decide they're going to be overweight and out of shape, a "heart attack waiting to happen." They don't wake up and hope they're clueless at relating to people, least of all close family members. And most don't set out to ignore God for years on end and then in times of crisis wonder why *he* seems so far away.

But these results happen untold thousands of times a day when people suddenly realize that changes need to be made or they are in danger of facing immediate consequences of a lifetime of bad choices.

If you decided to walk from San Francisco to Denver in a straight line but on your first day out veered off of that line by half a foot, where do you think you'd end up? A mathematician could tell you exactly, but you'd be in the neighborhood of Wyoming or New Mexico, depending on which direction you took. Maybe that would be close enough for you, but most people would wonder, *Now what?*

It's the "Now what?" as it relates to your life and health that this book wants to help answer. Because the truth is, nearly everyone has made that half-foot choice in the wrong direction in some area.

Everyone.

That's our nature. We can't help but slip off the path and then wish we'd taken another. The key isn't just realizing you've taken a rabbit trail to nowhere; it's getting back on the right trail to your desired destination.

That's the biggest reason the spiritual area of our life suddenly becomes the one place to begin (or continue) to take seriously. God specializes in helping his loved and unique creation to start over. We tell him where and when, and he's right there ready to help. His method of help isn't to transform our life like a fairy godmother would—waving a magic wand and making things all better. His method is first to draw us closer to himself and then to help us make decisions that will start developing the right characteristics in us.

And he doesn't leave us without the daily power to make the healthiest possible choices. As God knows, healthy choices make healthy people. We'll talk more about this aspect of the CREATION Health plan later on, but I want to give you hope that you won't have to be making choices completely under your own power. There's a power source just waiting for you to plug into.

SCIENTIFIC SUPPORT FOR CHOICE

Danish researchers led by Mette Andresen, PhD, examined the effect of freedom to make activity choices on the quality of life of nursing home residents. Their report found a positive effect, overall, when those studied perceived they had autonomy in these choices. Implications for changes in philosophy and delivery of nursing home care need further study.[1] The Andresen study followed up the much earlier findings of researchers Rodin and Langer, who examined how feeling free to choose affected the elderly, confined to a nursing home. The summary of their report says, "They selected two floors of a nursing home. One group was told the staff was there to help them. Despite the care, 71 percent got worse in only three weeks. In the other floor where they were encouraged to make decisions for themselves, the residents actually improved. They were more active and happier. They were more mentally alert and more active in activities."[2]

Regardless how old we are, when we make choices, we are taking responsibility and exerting a degree of control. This is a major determinant in how disease progresses. Scientist Dr. J. M. Koolhaas and his team found that even laboratory animals respond differently depending upon whether or not they are able to control their circumstances.[3] When exposed to adversity, animals that choose to stop the stress are far less likely to suffer from adverse effects compared with the animals that are helpless.[4] The same is true of people. Sometimes circumstances may leave little in your control. But you can always decide what you will focus upon and the attitude you adopt toward it.

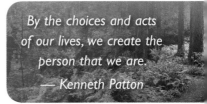

By the choices and acts of our lives, we create the person that we are.
— Kenneth Patton

For example, drugs that are used to manage chronic pain can become addictive. For that reason, physicians must carefully control and monitor the use of such drugs. However, researchers also discovered that patients grew anxious about whether medication would be available when needed, and this was actually making the pain worse for some patients. In a controversial decision, some hospitals allowed patients to administer their own pain medication whenever they needed it. Instead of using *more,* as expected, the patients actually took less medication.[5] Nothing new had been done to alleviate the pain, but now patients no longer worried about whether the nurse would hear their request or whether the drug would be made available. Just having the choice was enough to make the pain more tolerable.

TAKE CHARGE OF YOUR HEALTH

A few years ago, a young physician walked into Celebration Health— the "hospital of the twenty-first century." He was severely overweight and was starting to experience heart problems. Because his family had a history of heart disease, he was naturally concerned. He and his wife had just had a baby, and absolutely adoring his little girl, he wanted to be around to see her grow up.

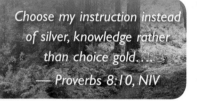

Choose my instruction instead of silver, knowledge rather than choice gold....
— Proverbs 8:10, NIV

When he started having heart symptoms, he decided, as a medical doctor, that it was time to take charge of his own health. So he came to our fitness center and started an exercise program. In time he lost more than forty pounds and began to change his entire health future.

One day at the fitness center I bumped into him. "Man!" I said. "You look totally different. What in the world's happened to you?"

"I've gotta tell you," he said. "One evening I had my little daughter crawl up in my lap. For the first time in my life I realized that I not only wanted to watch my children grow up but to see my grandchildren grow up as well. And I knew that if I was going to do that, I had to choose a different destiny than some of my other family members. I had to retain my health, and I had to make healthy choices.

"At first it was very hard work. But now it's become a lifestyle for me. I'm eating different, I'm living different, and I'm feeling different. And unless some freak accident happens, I believe that I will see my grandchildren and enjoy their company as well as I do my own children."

CHOICE GIVES HUMAN DIGNITY

Choice is our greatest asset and a very precious gift. Holocaust survivor Viktor E. Frankl wrote, "The last of human freedoms [is] . . . to choose one's own way."[6] Though he and his fellow prisoners could not control their environment, they could control their reactions, and Frankl observed that this choice often made the difference between survival and death, hopelessness and persecution.

Our ability to make decisions is one of the most important gifts that we human beings have. Ever notice how people feel hopeless when they don't have a choice? They feel like victims, that there is no point in trying to change their situation. Understanding that you do have a choice and that you always will, no matter what the circumstances, is a highly empowering thought. Therapists and counselors work hard to help clients see this truth; it's foundational to recovery.

How important are the choices we make?

Some choices, such as what color to wear to work, have no lasting consequences (unless your boss routinely fires people for wearing mauve). However, other decisions may result in outcomes that we have to live with for the rest of our lives. Studies show that many of the conditions we're dying from today—heart disease, hypertension, obesity, diabetes, and certain cancers—are the direct result of lifestyle choices. In many cases they are diseases of overeating and underactivity. Many of these diseases could be eliminated with healthier lifestyle choices.

When it comes to our physical health, our decisions do make a difference.

CHOICE IS A GIFT

God gave us choices from the very beginning, despite the fact that he knew that we might not always make the best ones.

In the Garden of Eden, Adam and Eve had a wealth of healthy options to choose from: fruits and vegetables to nourish them, physical work to strengthen their bodies, and a relationship with the Creator to feed their souls. But God also gave them another choice. "The Lord God took the man and put him in the Garden of Eden to work it and take care of it. And the Lord God commanded the man, 'You are free to eat from any tree in the garden; but you must not eat from the tree of the knowledge of good and evil, for when you eat of it you will surely die'" (Gen. 2:15–17).

That tree somehow represented all the unhealthy choices that Adam and Eve could make, all the decisions that could hurt them physically, spiritually, socially, and emotionally. Making this one choice—to eat from that tree—would result in a life that would be less than what God wanted for them. And in the end, the consequence would be twofold: physical death and separation from God—a short-term consequence and a very long-term consequence.

God didn't hide this choice from the first humans, nor did he pretend that it didn't exist. Instead, he lovingly created them as free moral agents with the ability to choose to follow his plan or choose to follow their own way. If you're a parent, then you know that the highest form of love you can have for your children, especially as they grow older, is to give them the freedom to choose their own way. It's the toughest thing a parent does, allowing their child to choose wisely or poorly, but it is absolutely necessary to protect the dignity of their lives.

Choice is at the very heart of God's wonderful plan for our health, both in this world and, of course, the next.

YOU HAVE A CHOICE

God loudly and clearly declares that he wants you to have a choice. And no matter your genetics or the condition of your environment, you can follow a healthy lifestyle. You can participate in your own healing, be part of the process of restoration. God has made you the steward of your own body. Do you recall that God still surrounded Adam and Eve with love even after they made unhealthy choices?

Look at what happened when they ate the forbidden fruit—when they began to realize what their decision would cost them and were overwhelmed with guilt. "And [Adam and Eve] heard the sound of the Lord God walking in the garden in the cool of the day, and Adam and his wife hid themselves from the presence of the Lord God among the trees of the garden" (Gen. 3:8, NKJV).

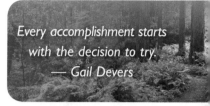

Every accomplishment starts with the decision to try.
— Gail Devers

Notice something rather amazing in this description. God himself was walking in the garden, looking for his children. Although he knew what had happened, he still wanted to continue the relationship. He didn't turn his back on them. The biblical account depicts Adam and Eve as the ones who were hiding. After he searched them out, God had to inform the couple about the consequences of their actions. But he also assured them that he still had a plan that would lead to life—he still had their best interest as his number-one priority.

GOOD CHOICES, GOOD INFORMATION

Managing your health is a challenge, one determined by the choices that you make daily. The Health Institute in Washington, DC, affirms that behavior change is related to a person's view of risk, benefit, and opportunity.[7] To make decisions that last, you must become more aware of your options and their consequences.[8] In this process, it is important to be honest with yourself. Ask the following questions:

- Do I really want change?

- Why is change so important for me now?

- What are all the benefits if I make smart health choices?

- What are the risks if I don't make good health choices?

One of the most important factors in making wise decisions is good information. The more you read and understand about your health, the more likely you are to be willing to change.

Sometimes knowledge is not enough, nor is sheer willpower. How often have you made New Year's resolutions that fizzle and die after only one month? David Katz, MD, MPH, of Yale School of Medicine, states that there has to be "a reasonable way" as well.[9] In other words, if the difficulty in making any changes outweighs your motivation, you will not alter your behavior. (We've all heard stories about people not using their health club memberships because the gym is all the way across town.)

The thought of making healthy changes can sound overwhelming, but it is not impossible. Choice is the foundation of a balanced, healthy life. The other seven CREATION Health principles will work only when we fully grasp our gift of choice and use it in concert with God's guidance.

> *The strongest principle of growth lies in the human choice.*
> — George Eliot

So what about it? Wouldn't you like to make healthy choices today? Right now you can start taking positive steps that will turn your life around—physically, spiritually, socially, and emotionally. Let me encourage you to decide every day to live the life for which God created you. You can begin a journey that will take you to a better place than you have ever imagined.

SUCCESS STEPS

Here are four practical steps to energize your *Choice* success:

CHOOSE—The first step to living a healthy, balanced life is to make the decision that it is what you want. Unless you're in the top 10 percent of the most disciplined people on the planet, it will be a daily choice, a commitment to live a balanced, healthy existence. Why not choose to read and follow a chapter of this book each week for eight life-changing weeks?

NOTICE—Once you have made the decision that God's prescription for living is the right choice, take a look at the balance of your life. Are there areas that are keeping you from enjoying full health? Which ones will you be able to bring into balance immediately? Which are best to hold off and call "long-term goals"?

PRIORITIZE—Look at the out-of-balance areas and choose your priorities. It would be wonderful if everything could be fixed at once, but it doesn't quite work that way. Choose one area (no more than two) for your attention. For example, if you are out of balance in the area of rest, what choices are you willing to make to increase your rest time? If your top priority is more activity, are you willing to get up early and take a walk? Healthy changes require conscious effort, so keep them simple and realistic. This will help to remove many barriers and set you up for success.

ACT—Having established your priorities, it's time to set goals and take action! Again, don't plan to bring everything into balance in a matter of hours. Instead, choose realistic small-step goals that you truly can do today. For instance, if your goal is to eat more healthfully, a goal of "never eating chocolate cake again" probably will not work. But choosing cake only once a week may be one good step on the road to nutritional success. Keep your goals simple and doable, and you will set yourself up for success.

Are you often in a hurry?

....

Do you get less than seven hours of sleep
per night?

....

Do you sometimes feel overwhelmed or
out of control?

....

Do small things cause you to have
big reactions?

....

Do you give the most important people in
your life undivided attention?

....

Do you need some ideas on how to find
more rest from your work?

....

The "R" in CREATION Health stands
for Rest.

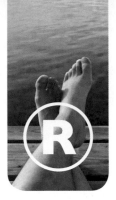

REST

CHAPTER 3

Getting Out of the Fast Lane

D O YOU KNOW THE WONDERFULLY SWEET PLEASURE of leaning back and reveling in a good rest? That's the gift God exemplified when he himself rested on the seventh day. And this seventh day of rest wasn't simply because he ran out of things to create. It was an intentional day that he ordained to send a message to us how essential rest is.

How can most of us learn the value of rest? The first way is to broaden our horizon on what rest truly can be.

Rest can come as a ten-minute power nap, a twenty-second mini-vacation, or eight hours of wonderful sleep. Regardless of its length, rest offers energy for the burned-out and restoration for the broken. Rest replaces weariness, exhaustion, and fatigue with peace, energy, and hope. Maybe that's why God showed us how important a whole day of rest could be. Knowing that we would work hard all week, he dedicated an entire day for us to plug into his power, a time when he would like to pack us full of himself so we can be healthier people throughout the next week.

Rest. It's God's personal way of saying, "Let's take some time together, just you and me."

SCIENTIFIC SUPPORT FOR REST

Researchers Bryant, Trinder, and Curtis found that the immune system is negatively affected when deprived of sleep. In other words, "…there is a reciprocal relationship between sleep and immunity. This relationship is important because, over recent decades, there has been a documented decrease in the mean duration and quality of sleep in the population."[10]

> *Come to me, all you who are weary and burdened, and I will give you rest.*
> — Jesus Christ

Much of this decrease is directly related to everyday stress. For every action there has to be an opposite and equal reaction. More than a law of physics, it's a requirement for optimal health. Stress is a part of daily living and not likely to go away. While you may have little influence over the circumstances that cause you anguish, you can insert periods of rest and recovery. Stress is beneficial in that it stimulates change and growth. However, it is during periods of recovery that the growth actually occurs. Successful athletes make recovery an essential part of their training, for without it, muscles will never achieve their full potential. In the same way, rest has to be your daily routine to protect you from illness. Rest and recovery balance out stress. Without this "R&R" you will never achieve optimal health.

While sleep comes to mind as a primary way to get our needed rest, there are other ways to rest apart from sleep. One of these is a relaxing massage. This type of rest could be more than just a quiet interlude from the topsy-turvy world you may live in. It can also be an essential ingredient for good health. Dr. Tiffany Field, at the University of Miami, demonstrated that premature infants who were gently massaged several times each day grew at a faster rate, developed reflexes more rapidly, and had cognitive advantages compared with those premature infants who were not touched.[11] Your skin is the largest organ in the body and, when touched, can release pain-countering endorphins as well as produce immune system-stimulating growth hormone.

Those seeking healing, not just pampering, are incorporating restful massages into their weekly schedules. Couples, of course, can do this for each other. Moms can give backrubs or foot massages to children and teens. There are many good books that teach techniques, but it doesn't take a pro to give a good massage. Just use long strokes and some kneading movements; add a little warm lotion or oil, and the recipient will be thankful . . . and delighted. It's that simple.

GETTING OUT OF THE FAST LANE

We are an overstimulated society.

The world around us seeks to cram more and more into each twenty-four-hour day. Businesses run at an ever-quickening pace. People phone, fax, e-mail, page, and overnight-deliver to us a flood of demands wherever we are in the world. And we have to respond in kind—just to keep up. And it's not just media overload we're affected by. Our schedules are jam-packed with great, kid-centered activities. There are more good things to be involved with than ever before, but must a family do all of them?

When we do sit down to relax, the stimulation only increases. Where once we had only thirteen television stations to choose from, today sixty to six hundred channels compete for our attention. And there are more on the way.

What about our night times?

Not much better.

According to Dr. James B. Maas of Cornell University, more than one hundred million Americans suffer from sleep deprivation.[12] More than 40 percent of Americans sleep less than six hours a night, and as many as one in three are so sleepy during the day that it interferes with their performance and activities at least two to three days in each month. And guess what? Stress is the number one cause for poor sleep. Consider these familiar scenarios:

A stock trader exchanges a full night's sleep for fitful naps between transactions as he frantically tries to follow market activity around the world.

A young mother accepts the night shift so she can take care of her children during the day. She describes her world as exhausting and speaks of sleep with the craving of a hungry beggar talking about food. But as she works what is basically an eighty-hour week, she risks her health, her sanity, and her marriage. As she chases her dream of the good life, it cruelly imprisons her with a sentence of hard labor.

THE NEMO SYNDROME—A FISH STORY

Tony and Sonya Nicholson donated two beautiful aquariums to a local hospital. It completely changed the atmosphere in the lobby. Instead of an unknown, unfriendly environment that intimidated children, it was immediately transformed to a place of delight. The brilliant clown fish particularly attracted young kids. You could hear them squeal, "Look, Mommy, it's Nemo!"

But within a week, the fish began dying. Every few days "Nemo" had

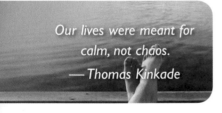

Our lives were meant for calm, not chaos.
— Thomas Kinkade

to be replaced. The staff called in the aquarium experts, but they couldn't find the problem either. Finally one of them asked, "Are the lights always on in this area of the hospital?" The answer was yes. "Maybe that's the problem," he replied. "They aren't getting any darkness for rest." So every night the staff turned off the aquarium light. And the result? Nemo lived!

An overstimulated world of beepers, cell phones, TVs, radios, and music players could give you the "Nemo syndrome." No time for proper rest could put you in an early grave. The solution: seven hours of sleep at night, quiet time with God in the morning, pause at lunch to pray, and one day a week off to celebrate love—a weekly sabbatical to refresh your song.

FINDING THE BALANCE

With each beat, our hearts teach us the importance of respecting natural rhythms—the necessity to balance work and rest. Should you live to age seventy, during your lifetime your heart will beat 2.5 billion times and will pump more than one million barrels of blood throughout your body. It is important to note that between each powerful beat of your heart, it rests. This resting period allows the heart to reload—to do the work of the next beat.

Likewise, you and I need time to "reload." We need rest. The medical community understands this principle well—every day they see its effects when ignored. Overstimulated organs eventually flatline. That means they shut down and die.

Kathy, a cardiac lab nurse, compares our need for rest to the heart rhythm itself. "When we take care of patients," Kathy says, "we always give them an electrocardiogram [EKG], an electrical recording of the heart. It shows us the heart rhythm, or heartbeat, which is the very basis of what we do. I like to compare the heartbeat to how God made us. Each waveform is a heartbeat, and the line that separates each beat is a time of rest. This is the way our lives work as well. We can have a very active day, and then we need a time of rest. We need sleep in order to stay healthy."

Kathy says they're constantly trying to teach their cardiac patients how to take time every day for rest, relaxation, and rejuvenation. And what about those who are going through emotional turmoil? Though they may not appear active, people suffering from tragedy or loss will feel exhausted and need more sleep. Grief is work, and our body seems to know it needs rest in the draining periods of life. Quakers have a process called "centering down." It refers to a calm stillness within . . . a restful place we can feel and go to, with practice, when life gets off-kilter.

God has placed the rhythm of rest within the very pulse of your own body by giving rest in each heartbeat, in each day, and in each week. Why not step out of the fast lane and enjoy some sweet rest?

THE REST ZONE

In our stressed-out world, in which families are increasingly falling apart and thousands visit hospital emergency rooms each day because their stress has become a major health crisis, we desperately need the kind of rest that God offers. Here is my paraphrase of the invitation Jesus made in Matthew 11:28: "Come unto me all you who labor to exhaustion, and I will give you rest."

HeartMath is an organization begun by a group of scientists dedicated to teaching people how to gain maximum health through getting the circulatory, respiratory, and nervous systems back into sync. Their approach is to teach simple activities you can do right now to bring your body back into balance.

HeartMath urges us to take power breaks; as little as five minutes will make a tremendous difference in how you feel and how well your body works. Breathe deeply, relax your mind with peaceful thoughts, and pray. Such breaks will have profound impact on your body and your performance.[13] Research shows that when we are in sync, blood pressure drops, stress hormones plummet, anti-aging hormones increase, clarity and calmness result.[14]

In short, you experience the benefits of rest. This is especially important when you face a crisis. It will enable you to be your best. Athletes call this being "in the zone"—the rest zone! You find out more about this amazing approach to rest on the Internet at *HeartMath.com*.

YOU DESERVE A SABBATICAL

Science, however, wasn't the first to discover the need for a cycle of rest. In fact, rest is part of the plan that God gave to us at the very beginning. He established an island of time at the end of each week for spiritual and physical restoration.

The book of Genesis tells how God provided for this rest. During a six-day period, God created all the living things on our planet, everything from crickets to crocodiles, from mushrooms to mangoes. He also made the first human beings.

It was an amazing week of work, and God knew it. "God saw all that he had made, and it was very good" (Gen. 1:31). Everything was good indeed. We're still discovering today the awe-inspiring ways in which he designed even the tiniest of creatures—living things so small we can view them only through powerful microscopes.

But then watch what happened: "Thus the heavens and the earth were completed in all their vast array. By the seventh day God had finished the work he had been doing; so on the seventh day he rested from all his work" (Gen. 2:1–2).

What was God doing here? Was he worn out from his work?

Not likely. Instead he was exemplifying and building a rhythm of rest into our weekly cycle. This cycle is as much a part of nature as the rhythm of our hearts: beat, rest, beat, rest. God was creating an island of rest in our ocean of labor.

He would make that clear when he gave the world the familiar Ten Commandments from Mount Sinai. Among these basic moral principles is one that prescribes rest. The fourth commandment reads: "Remember the Sabbath day, to keep it holy. Six days you shall labor and do all your work, but the seventh day is the Sabbath of the Lord your God. In it you shall do no work" (Ex. 20:8–10, NKJV).

In other words, God is saying: "Great news! You don't have to work this day, and you don't have to feel guilty about it. This is a day for resting."

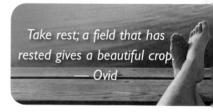

Take rest; a field that has rested gives a beautiful crop.
— Ovid

By the way, notice something else interesting about the weekly cycle of activity and rest. The seven-day week is the only part of our calendars that doesn't correspond to some celestial cycle. Think about it.

We have the year, the time it takes the earth to orbit the sun. We have the month, the period from one full moon to the next. And we have the twenty-four-hour day, the time it takes the earth to rotate once on its axis.

But the week? Where does that come from? Nature has no seven-day cycles that repeat themselves again and again. Yet virtually everyone on earth observes a seven-day week.

Why?

The week was given to everyone by the hand of God. Going back to the beginning, it's a direct link through time to the One who fashioned life on our planet. And at the climax of that week, God rested. He set aside a day to experience love—a practice that will bring you health.

DISCOVERING TRUE REST

Rest, of course, can come in many forms—through sleep, through relaxation, through meditation, through prayer, through worship, and even through relationships. Mainly I've found that true rest comes through a divine person— and that person is Jesus Christ. Others are also discovering that same fact.

Scott: From Stress to Rest

Scott Brady, MD, a physician who uses the CREATION Health principles in his medical practice, tells of his personal journey from stress to rest.

"My wife and I had been married about five years," Dr. Brady says. "Things were going well, and we had our first child. I was studying for boards, and both of us were working full-time. Then I began to develop some physical symptoms—back pain, headaches, and stomach problems. Medicines weren't able to help. I saw about six or seven physicians, had several different diagnoses, lots of X-rays, physical therapy. And it kept getting worse to the point at which I was having about ten shots in my back every couple weeks just to be able to stand. I could sleep only two or three hours a night.

"It was really affecting our family. Soon I began to realize that it was more than just pain—that there were other things behind it: stresses and emotions I hadn't recognized. Once I began to acknowledge the emotions that were building up in me like a volcano, the pain started to go away. God became increasingly important in my life as I saw that I needed him more and more. I needed to rest in his grace."

As Scott discovered, sometimes chronic pain and illness aren't the result of genetics or physical factors but have their roots in emotional or spiritual problems. Recognizing these problems is the first step toward finding the rest that God intends for each of us. To learn more about Dr. Brady's story and how he has helped countless patients overcome chronic pain, including back pain, migraines, fibromyalgia, sciatica, irritable bowel syndrome, insomnia, and many others—see his book *Pain Free for Life: The 6-Week Cure for Chronic Pain without Surgery or Drugs.*[15]

Anxiety and fear are the opposite of rest. Life is filled with challenges from financial problems to personality conflicts. These challenges confront you at home, work, and in social situations. They can wear you out physically, mentally, and spiritually. You need to be free from these burdens. You need emotional rest as well as physical rest. This is why God invites you to put all your care on him, and he will give you rest.

> *True silence is the rest of the mind; it is to the spirit what sleep is to the body, nourishment and refreshment.*
> — Sir William Penn

Steve: Finding Space in My Life

A successful, young attorney named Steve noticed his hectic schedule was taking its toll on his health.

"I was leading a very, very busy life—sometimes putting in seventy-hour weeks," he explains. "Every month or so I had a pretty bad migraine. I was in my early thirties and had never had migraines before. My life had just gotten so busy, and I was so tired, that some cracks and strains were beginning to show in my relationships, including the one with my wife.

"I started to pray and to try to analyze my life and figure out what was missing. One of the first things that hit me was my schedule. I didn't have any time for rest. To me, rest is space within my life—space to step back and to reconnect with God, with my family, with my friends.

Rest is time to recharge my batteries and restore my enthusiasm with life and people. I really just needed to find that space in my life.

> Finish each day before you begin the next, and interpose a solid wall of sleep between the two.
> — Ralph Waldo Emerson

"I began making sure I got quality time with God. That happens both in the morning as well as on my Sabbath day of rest. The greatest benefit for me is that by increasing the amount of rest in my life, I'm now living more of a reflective life than a reactive one. Rather than a knee-jerk reaction to my circumstances, I take more time to determine what's really important to me."

Thousands of people like Scott and Steve are discovering that spiritual rest is a key part of healthy living. Taking time to bond with God creates a peaceful center in our lives. And it's from that peaceful center that we can grow toward wholeness.

RATING YOUR REST HABITS – A SELF-SURVEY

Sometimes life seems to dictate our pace instead of the reverse, and before we know it we're running nonstop, like Scott and Steve. If you can identify with them, you may find it helpful to use the following survey to evaluate your current rest habits. Just check each box that applies. There are no right or wrong answers; it's just a way to "see" yourself on paper, which can guide you toward making changes if you need to do so.

I have to jump-start my brain in the morning and/or afternoon with:

- ☐ Caffeine *(coffee, tea, soda, other)*
- ☐ Sugar *(doughnuts, candy, chocolate, etc.)*
- ☐ Medication

More often than I wish, I find it difficult to concentrate. When this happens, I:

- ☐ Take a nap

☐ Take a brisk walk

☐ Slog my way through it

I often find myself:

☐ Multitasking *(driving, eating, talking on phone—all at same time)*

☐ Overcommitting *(trying to cram too many things into a day)*

☐ Being crisis driven *(other people or events running my life; it is out of control)*

☐ Being too emotional *(overreacting to small things)*

Sometimes during the day I feel:

☐ Worried and unable to relax my mind

☐ Anxious about things I can't always identify

☐ Panic, like things are spinning out of control

My typical experience with sleep is that:

☐ I don't get enough sleep

☐ I don't sleep deeply

☐ I can't sleep

☐ I almost never wake up feeling rested

In terms of my work:

☐ I work sixty or more hours a week, including work I bring home

☐ I feel guilty for neglecting my family, but I must work to pay the bills

☐ When someone else suggests that my life is out of balance, I agree, but I also feel trapped

Honestly, what does this survey tell you about yourself?

Is there anything you would change if you could? Use the following success steps to guide your thinking.

SUCCESS STEPS

Here are seven practical steps toward incorporating *REST* into your healthy living strategy:

PRAY—Worry and anxiety often stand between us and real rest and health. Instead of becoming upset while waiting in traffic, talk with God. When you've had a rough day at work, tell him. Let him know your worries and cares. Then turn them over to him and trust that he will take care of you. The Bible tells us in Philippians 4:6–7: "Do not be anxious about anything, but in everything, by prayer and petition, with thanksgiving, present your requests to God. And the peace of God, which transcends all understanding, will guard your hearts and your minds in Christ Jesus."

SLEEP—Develop a regular sleep pattern. If you are sleeping less than seven to eight hours nightly, you are cheating yourself. Trying to catch up on sleep doesn't help. Here's how to get those restful zzz's: exercise daily; reduce caffeine intake, especially late in the day; reduce alcohol; avoid eating large, fatty meals late in the day that can keep you awake; adopt a relaxing bedtime routine, something that prepares you for sleep, such as a warm bubble bath or listening to soft music.

BREATHE WELL—Proper breathing can help you relax. Try this: start from the very bottom of your lungs and breathe in slowly through your nose. Count slowly to five while inhaling. Then exhale through tight lips twice as long as you inhaled. Allow the head to drop toward the chest as you exhale, relaxing the back of your neck. Repeat this exercise four or five times until you notice your breathing is slowing down. Explore other breathing techniques.

IMAGINE—Take twenty-second (or much longer!) mental vacations. Wander through Yosemite National Park, walk along a white-sand Hawaiian beach, or browse in antique shops in Pennsylvania. By taking time "away" you will resettle or "re-sync" your mind and be able to face your day with new energy.

TAKE A VACATION—We all love vacations but hardly ever take them. The average American worker feels that his workload just doesn't allow for the luxury of a vacation. It is no wonder that we are living unhealthy, unbalanced lives because a balanced, healthy life includes regular time off. No, not just an occasional day here and there—even though those are helpful—but the "I went fishing in the Keys for two weeks" kind of vacations. Studies show that our bodies need several days to unwind from the stress of everyday life. Then we need several days after that for true rest to occur. Start planning your next vacation, a real one, without cell phones, computers, and other work. Get away. Play. Rest.

LAUGH—The book of Proverbs in the Bible tells us that a cheerful heart is good medicine, but a crushed spirit dries up the bones. Another way of saying this is that laughter is the best medicine. When we laugh, especially those laughs that start in our toes and don't stop until they reach the top of our head, our blood pressure goes down, our muscles relax, and our brain releases chemicals (endorphins) that make us feel better. You can add laughter to your life in countless ways. Keep a joke or riddle book handy. Watch reruns of *I Love Lucy, The Dick van Dyke Show,* or *The Three Stooges.* Keep a funny video collection (it's cheaper than therapy). Go to a local pet store and watch the kittens and puppies play. Find whatever makes you laugh, then do it!

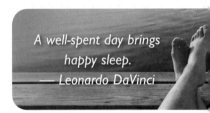

A well-spent day brings happy sleep.
— Leonardo DaVinci

REST WEEKLY—Never forget the special Sabbath rest that God created for us. The word "Sabbath" comes from the Hebrew word transliterated shabath (to cease or to rest). When we leave behind our normal routine and spend a full day with him and with family and friends, it's amazing how ready we are to tackle another week. Spend portions of this day reading the Bible and praying, enjoying nature, visiting a nursing home, going to church. Keep some devotional books handy and learn to journal. Rest your body, your mind, and your soul.

Is your life filled with too much noise?

....

Do you ever wish you could create a
peaceful space somewhere to escape to?

....

Do you feel stressed by the constant
changes life throws your way?

....

Would you like to know a secret for
uncluttering your thoughts?

....

Do you know how to express your need
for human touch?

....

Do you know how much your environment
affects your health?

....

The "E" in CREATION Health stands
for Environment.

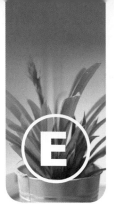

ENVIRONMENT

CHAPTER 4

Practicing the Principles of Paradise

GOD DESIGNED THE WORLD TO PERFECTLY MATCH the people who would live in it. Then he handed it to us and said, "Take good care of it—for me."

As caretakers, we've discovered a special healing relationship between people and nature. Dig in your garden and be energized. Plant a row of petunias on your windowsill and be amazed. Watch a five-minute sunset and be revitalized.

We can find healing in a robin's song or in walking beside the sea. There is healing on a mountain trail, in the desert sands, in a pine forest, on a rocky coast, and in a city park. Nature brings healing to the body, mind, and spirit. God made it that way.

SCIENTIFIC SUPPORT FOR ENVIRONMENT

You probably have heard of Pavlov and his dogs. After allowing them to smell food while listening to a bell, he discovered that the bell alone soon induced salivation. The same thing can happen in your body. Just about anything in the environment can elicit an automatic response after an association has been established. Cancer patients, upon returning to the clinic where they received chemotherapy, will sometimes re-experience the side effects of the treatment even though they do not get any medication. Instead, pictures in the room, the fragrance worn by a staff member, and even the background music are responsible. This research, conducted at the Sloan Kettering Memorial Hospital in New York, underscores why it is essential to pay attention to anything at home or work that may affect your health. You may not make the connection, but your body can.[16]

> *God almighty first planted a garden: and, indeed, it is the purest of human pleasure.*
> — *Francis Bacon*

We all remember where we were and what we were doing when we heard of the attack on the World Trade Towers in New York City. Those who were there will do more than remember. The slightest reminder may trigger the same stress response they experienced during the attack. In the extreme, it results in a condition called *post traumatic stress disorder*, or PTSD. Scientists have shown that the more emotion associated with an event, the more likely it will leave a permanent memory in your brain. We live among triggers of both unhealthy and healthy responses. Positive emotions will do the same thing. That's why we remember our wedding day or the first time we got up on a slalom ski. For optimal health, create an environment that will remind you of the positive while removing those things that might trigger anxiety.

CONSTANT CHANGE, CONTINUAL STRESS

Today we live in a world of never-ending changes in styles. The latest fashions, fads, and trends grow faster and fall flatter than ever before. All around us billboards, radio, television, magazines, the Internet, and more shout for our time and attention and beg to be noticed. As a result, many feel as though their lives are growing ever more stressful as they try to keep up with the constant changes.

Medical scientists are highlighting today that our environment has a significant impact on our health.

THE EDEN ENVIRONMENT

Take a moment to think about your personal environment—both at home and in your workplace. Are your surroundings cheerful and healthy? Are they places that nurture your soul and recharge your spirit? Do you feel calm and happy when you're in them? Do they provide you with comfort, offer you an opportunity for growth, and give you a sense of peace?

God knew the effect our environment would have on us. That's why he placed the first humans in the best possible surroundings. Though we can't expect to recreate the Garden of Eden, we can take principles away from it and then apply them to our own situations— enriching our homes and enlivening our workplaces by lessons learned from the natural world.

Let's examine the Eden environment to see what we can discover for our use today.

SIGHT SENSE: A PLACE OF PEACE

Scenes of God's handiwork surrounded Adam and Eve in Eden. I can envision awesome trees, fragrant flowers, babbling brooks, majestic mountains, and peaceful ponds. And in all of God's work, order and simplicity prevailed.

Take a critical look at your personal environment. Are simplicity and order the rule or the exception? After a routine cleaning of your home, does it still feel cluttered? Stacks of old magazines scattered about? Closets stuffed with clothes you rarely or never wear? Too many appliances crowding your kitchen counter space? Whether we realize it or not, the very sight of clutter saps our energy, drains our strength, and depletes our sense of peace.

As curious as it may sound, many people have found that by uncluttering their environment they begin to free their thoughts, their emotions, and even their priorities. A simple, clean environment helps to clear your mind and create a greater sense of peace.

To establish a sense of visual warmth in your home, display objects that awaken good memories. Surround yourself with things that bring a feeling of peace, comfort, and joy. Perhaps your treasures are pictures of family and friends—or awards or honors that you've earned and received. Art may bring you energy: paintings full of color or sculptures brimming with life. Display items that remind you to dream—that draw you to God.

Before his death, Henri Matisse, the great modern French painter, spent many months bedridden with colon cancer. His family moved his bed so he could take in the view of the countryside from the bedroom window. More importantly, they kept changing what was on his windowsill so he could be continually inspired to paint. Some of his most famous pieces were painted from his deathbed.

> Nobody can be in good health if he does not have all the time, fresh air, sunshine, and good water.
> — Chief Flying Hawk, Oglala Sioux

Why not take a cue from the Matisse family? Add a little visual spice to your space. Try rotating or alternating your family photos, artwork, and displays. Many picture frames now hold several pictures at once, so you can change the subjects often. You can also treat them as a traveling art show by shifting them from room to room. Or you might consider an electronic picture frame, into which you can load and show your favorite photos, in effect creating an ever-changing slide show. A change of location also works well with plants. Besides being aesthetically pleasing, the visual variety may inspire you to new levels of personal creativity—as it did for Henri Matisse.

Another way to add visual zest to your personal space is to let the sunshine in. Open the blinds, draw back the curtains, throw open the shutters, and let the natural light pour in. Sunlight has many benefits—among them the ability to cheer you by brightening your personal space. A lighter home is often a brighter home.

In their book *Health Power: Healthy by Choice, Not by Chance*, Aileen Ludington and Hans Diehl suggest that sunlight has a lot to offer.[17]

In proper amounts it enhances the immune system, alleviates pain from swollen arthritic joints, relieves certain premenstrual symptoms, and lowers blood cholesterol levels. Sunlight can lift your spirits, improve your sleep, and increase your energy. Consult your doctor or dermatologist about how to enjoy the benefits of sunlight safely.

As you strive to make your personal environment a little piece of paradise, pay attention to the visuals that surround you. Clear away the clutter and move toward simplicity. You'll find that the loss is really a gain.

SMELL SENSE: MAKING GOOD SCENTS

Scents have become big business. From supermarkets and drugstores to department stores and boutiques, everyone seems to be getting into the trade of selling good scents. But which is the right scent for you?

A good place to start is to head back to the garden. What did God do to enhance the sense of smell in Eden? For one thing, he filled it with plants—all sorts of plants. Considering that more than 55,000 species of flowering plants grow in the Amazon rain forest, just imagine what Eden might have been like. Flowering and nonflowering plants. Leafy plants. Creeping plants. Water plants and land plants. Such an enormous variety. Of course, they were beautiful to look at, but they also cleaned the air.

So take a tip from God and place plenty of plants in your personal space. When you do, you'll be increasing the quality of the air you breathe (scientific research from NASA has shown that foliage and flowering plants help purify the air).[18] Sure, it takes a little work, but the rewards are great.

Beyond flowers and plants, try other creative methods to make your space more fragrant. One way is to light the scented candles you find available in specialty shops, grocery stores, department stores, and pharmacies. Here are just a few of the many scents available—and what they can do for you:

Eucalyptus clears the head and invigorates the mind.

Chamomile is said to bring relaxation.

Pine is thought to stimulate creativity.

Orange is supposed to refresh the mind.

Tea tree is said to ground your thoughts.

Thyme is believed to refresh and strengthen the immune system.

Cucumber is thought to calm the nerves.

Find a few scents that you enjoy, and bring them home to try. You'll be wonderfully pleased with the tranquil frame of mind they help create.

Still other ways exist to freshen the scent of your environment, including: aromatherapy kits, potpourri pots, air freshener plug-ins, room sprays, car deodorizing trees, bubble baths, body lotions, and scented oils. And don't forget about the perfume or cologne you wear. It can be a great way to share your good scents. Then there's the kitchen. Bread baking, corn cooking, soup simmering—fabulous smells from the kitchen can wake up and warm our souls.

Discover what fragrances are your favorites—and surround yourself with them.

SOUND SENSE: TUNE IN TO LIFE'S NATURAL RHYTHMS

A day spent in nature is a day surrounded by sound. The playful rustle of wind dancing through trees. The soothing coos of a mourning dove. The ceaseless rhythm of the ocean. The enchanting chirp of crickets on a summer's eve. Swirling water tumbling over itself in a lively brook. The peaceful patter of rain on leafy trees. Thunder rumbling across the sky. Nature is a veritable symphony of sound. And God is its great conductor.

Back in the garden, Adam and Eve became accustomed to living by the natural rhythms of life.

They had no clocks, so they rose with the sun and slept with the stars—the natural rhythm of a day.

They worked six days and rested on the seventh—the natural rhythm of a week.

They grew and gathered food—the natural rhythm of seasons.

They had no radios or audio players, so their music was the melody of nature—the natural rhythm of sound.

In contrast to the soothing sounds of Eden, the average office today is likely to be filled with the constant drone of ringing phones, beeping pagers, and whining fax machines. And out of the office, you and I will encounter honking traffic, blaring radios, noisy malls, and endlessly chattering televisions. The constant clamor can make it difficult to clear our minds and think.

"In twentieth-century society," comments Steven Halpern, contemporary musician, "the noise level is such that it keeps knocking our bodies out of tune and out of their natural rhythms. This ever-increasing assault of sound upon our ears, minds, and bodies adds to the stress load of civilized beings trying to live in a highly complex environment."[19]

Artist Luigi Russolo observed that "in antiquity there was only silence. In the nineteenth century, with the invention of the machine, noise was born. Today, noise triumphs and reigns supreme."[20]

> The Lord God took the man and put him in the Garden of Eden to work it and take care of it.
> — *Genesis 2:15, NIV*

The Garden of Eden, a place of perfect peace, stands in striking contrast to the modern world of manufactured noise. What can we do to save our sanity? Let's explore three possible alternatives to the increasing assault of sound on our personal environments.

SILENCE. In a noisy, clamoring, overstimulated society, silence seems like a lost art. Indeed, many have become so accustomed to noise that they actually feel uncomfortable in silence. Some even prefer to fall asleep at night with the television or radio on. British poet

Dame Edith Sitwell once remarked, "My personal hobbies are reading, listening to music, and silence."[21] Sometimes the best thing you can do is to shut out sound of every kind and sit in silence. Somewhere in the silence you may find it easier to tune in to God's voice as he speaks to you of his love.

NATURAL RHYTHMS. To restore a sense of peace and harmony to your home (or workplace), consider filling it with sounds from nature—the natural rhythms designed by God to bring rest to the spirit. You might start by looking into nature recordings. Many companies offer high-quality recordings of nature sounds for your enjoyment: ocean waves, gurgling brooks, gentle rain, waterfalls, wind through the trees, birds in song, and the many voices of the rain forest. Some artists have set these soothing sounds to relaxing instrumental music. Find out which ones help you to relax.

> Experiencing nature is an important pathway to human health and well-being....The more technology we embrace, the more nature we need.
> — CREATION Health Life Guide - You Were Made For a Garden

Inexpensive sound generators are also widely available today. They generate natural sounds to help drown out unwanted background noise. If you happen to live in a noisy city or next to a heavily trafficked road, you might find a sound generator useful. They can often reproduce the rhythms of rain, waterfalls, rivers, and the beating of ocean surf. If you're a pet lover, you may want to consider owning a songbird. Another restful sound is that of a tabletop fountain—and, of course, fountains are also enjoyable to watch.

RELAXING MUSIC. Music, it's been said, is simply noise that someone has organized. Many studies suggest that music has a calming effect on the human body and mind. Listening to soothing music may reduce stress, decrease muscle tension, strengthen the immune system, raise endorphin levels, and produce feelings of peace. No one kind of music soothes and relaxes everyone. Many enjoy the piano, flute, guitar, or harp. Others prefer classical music or smooth jazz. Discover the style that makes you feel relaxed and at peace. Then keep it handy when stress starts to rise.

TASTE SENSE: TANTALIZE YOUR TASTE BUDS NATURALLY

When it came to food in the Garden of Eden, Adam and Eve ate like the king and queen they were, for the God who made them provided what was best for them. Everything they needed for perfect health was right there in the garden.

Genesis 1:29 gives us the basic description: "Then God said, 'I give you every seed-bearing plant on the face of the whole earth and every tree that has fruit with seed in it. They will be yours for food.'" It was a simple yet wonderful menu.

The original human diet, as designed by God himself, was to be one consisting of fruits, vegetables, grains, and nuts. And every bite was a delight. Adam and Eve had the most delicious berries, the ripest apples, the juiciest oranges, the plumpest plums, the tastiest nuts, the freshest grains, the yellowest squash, the best potatoes, the sweetest tomatoes, and the crunchiest cucumbers. In addition, they had the purest water for refreshment. It was all theirs for the choosing.

Tasting the treasures of nature is one of God's greatest gifts. Eating may be a necessity, but enjoying the experience is not. Yet God in his goodness gave us pleasure in food. Of course, some food choices are better than others. And our modern track record has not been so good.

Often we substitute sugary snacks for the sweetness of fruit. We trade the goodness of vegetables for fatty fast foods. Many of us swap the vitality of pure water for sweetened syrupy drinks. As a result, we exchange healthy nutrition for empty calories. The result is taste buds that become accustomed to the assault of sugars, fats, and nutrition-free foods. It's no wonder that so many people find little pleasure in natural eating plans.

Even when we do try to eat a healthy diet, too many of us don't take the time to enjoy it. Busy people with hectic lives grab a meal on the run—one hand on our food, the other on our work. Or we eat while being entertained, diminishing the actual meal experience.

Would you like to try an experiment? Tonight for dinner, actually sit at a table while not allowing any outside distractions: no TV, no phone, no newspaper, no mail, no work assignments. Take the time to really look at your food. Notice all the colors and textures. You can even listen as you eat for the sounds that it creates. Relish the texture of the food in your mouth. Savor the smells. Take in the tastes. Don't rush through the meal with your thoughts on what you have to do next. God gave you the sense of taste to enhance your life. Enjoy it! Let every bite be a delight.

TOUCH SENSE: THRIVING THROUGH THE GENTLE TOUCH

Would an all-powerful God ever create something that was incomplete? Unfinished? Not whole? Apparently so. Seems rather hard to believe, but in the midst of perfection something was found lacking—like a bare patch of canvas on an artist's finished masterpiece. But there it was—God's unfinished business.

In the Genesis account of Creation, God made the earth in just seven days. At the end of each day, he stood back to examine his handiwork. For five days in a row his assessment was the same: "And God saw that it was good." But on the sixth day something unusual occurred. For the first time he said that part of Creation was "not good." Here's the exact quote from Genesis 2:18: "The Lord God said, 'It is not good for the man to be alone. I will make a helper suitable for him.'"

After his wondrous work in creating Adam, the first man, God recognized that something was amiss. The human being needed a partner. A life mate. A love mate. Someone to hold his hand as he walked through the garden. Someone to slip his arm around as the sun sank into the west. Someone to snuggle with as the stars came out. Someone to have and to hold for a lifetime. And so God created

Eve. She was Adam's equal in every way. Together they were to rule the world—in love with God and in love with each other.

What was true at Creation is still so today—people need others to survive and thrive. We each require helpmates and heart mates to make it through life. One of the ways we can aid each other to flourish is through the wonderful gift of touch. The skin God created for each of us is the largest sense organ in our bodies and responds positively to every loving touch.

Numerous studies document the fact that we must have touch to develop and grow.[22] Research has shown that women who are hugged regularly tend to live longer and have fewer heart problems.[23]

In his classic book *Psychosocial Medicine: A Study of the Sick Society*, James L. Halliday wrote that infants deprived of regular maternal body contact can develop profound depression with an accompanying lack of appetite and wasting so severe that it can lead to death.[24]

> *To sit in the shade on a fine day, and look upon verdure is the most perfect refreshment.*
> — *Jane Austen*

In modern healthcare we have to take precautions to prevent the spread of infections. Therefore, the hand is covered with a glove, and a synthetic touch replaces the touch of skin. The mask covers a sympathetic smile, and glasses shield the eyes. We would love to be able to communicate our care skin-to-skin, but it would violate the roles of modern healthcare. This is why it is even more important that you touch your loved ones and hold them close. We are healed as we are touched. It's God's original design, and it still works today.

Somewhere deep in the fabric of the human heart God placed a desire to love and be loved. Touch and be touched. Well-known family therapist Virginia Satir once stated that we need four hugs a day for survival, eight a day for maintenance, and twelve a day for growth.[25] How do you express your need for human contact? Do you have someone you can turn to for a soothing word and a gentle touch? If not, one of the best ways to find such a friend is to be that kind of friend to others.

We can also enjoy our God-given sense of touch through the textures around us. Velvety pillows and rough burlap. Silky clothes and coarse carpeting. Smooth grass and sharp stones. All are sensations we experience through the sense of touch. In your personal environment have you taken the time to surround yourself with things you like to feel?

> It's a feeling of awe . . . this feeling about the glories of the universe.
> — Richard Feynman

Are there fluffy pillows to caress your head as you snuggle into bed? Do you have a favorite overstuffed chair you can flop into and relax? Is your home carpeting gentle on the feet? Do you wear comfortable clothing that's soft on the skin? The next time you go shopping, try a different approach. Rather than simply searching for the latest styles, try feeling the fabric first. Run your hand down the clothing rack or over the shelves until you find something pleasant to the touch. Only then should you pull it out and take a look at the style. If you need extra guidance, ask a sales attendant for help in finding natural fiber fabric. The softer texture is sure to be a sensory explosion next to your skin. You might be surprised how much better you feel in clothing chosen for comfort rather than chic.

Take some time this week to explore creative ways you can make your personal environment a more touching place to be.

WHEN YOU CAN'T CHANGE THINGS

You may struggle with limitations on how much you can alter your environment, especially in the workplace. Not everyone wants your "soothing music" floating into their ears—not to mention your pet songbird's chirping. When you can't quite attain Eden-like beauty on the outside, try doing it within.

A few years ago, a hospital nurse was getting frustrated with an old copy machine that produced copies very slowly. On one particular occasion, while waiting for her job to finish, she decided she wasn't going to let it frustrate her—she would use that time to pray. She made a particular request to the Lord—and her prayer received an answer. The next time she made copies, she prayed again. And again. "Over a period of time," she said, "I found myself in front of that machine, taking more and more requests to the Lord." And she kept getting positive responses.

When she shared her experience with some of her fellow workers, they started doing the same thing. It got to the point where they began keeping a list of the requests and the date on which the Lord had answered the prayer. Soon they went from despising that old copy machine to treasuring it.

So even if it seems you can't change your environment for the better, you can change your perspective and thereby your experiences of it.

"Do not be conformed to this world, but be transformed by the renewing of your mind, that you may prove what is that good and acceptable and perfect will of God" (Rom. 12:2, NKJV).

Your environment influences your health. As often as you can, establish one that fosters peace and well-being. Remember the importance of fresh air and sunlight. Try to have a home situation that allows you to relax. And if this is out of your control, create a restful room, a quiet nook, or an Eden-like space in your backyard (the Japanese have practiced this secret for centuries). Remember the benefits of sight and aromatherapy. Enjoy both music and silence. Choose to take time with your meals. And never forget the wonderfully healthy benefit of hugging and embracing those you love.

SUCCESS STEPS

Here are five practical steps to energize your *ENVIRONMENT* success:

SIGHT—Add beautiful sights to your personal world. Place a plant on your office desk. Add a bouquet of flowers to the kitchen table. Hang a calendar or other photographs of nature on a wall you look at often. Buy a low-maintenance betta fish and make friends with it. Watch a sunset.

SOUND—Change your environment by adding peaceful sounds to your life. Get a tabletop fountain and listen to the flowing water. Purchase a nature sound generator and relax to the rhythm of falling rain or ocean waves. Get a pet songbird and listen to it sing. Discover a style of music that makes you feel relaxed and at peace, then put it on when you feel stressed. If you haven't tried classical music before, pick up a copy of one of these favorites: Pachelbel's "Canon in D," Beethoven's "Moonlight Sonata," or Debussy's "Claire de Lune." Also remember, sometimes complete silence is the best remedy for an overstimulated day.

TOUCH—Use touch every day to lead a happier, more aware life. Reach out for a friend's arm when engaged in conversation. Ask for and give appropriate hugs. Choose clothing that feels good on you, not just that looks good. Pamper yourself and have a massage. Take a hot bath at the end of a long day.

TASTE—Be adventurous! Eat a variety of colors—yellow, orange, brown, red, and green. Find a farmer's market near you and get lots of fresh fruits and veggies to eat. Choose crunchy, whole-grain breads and cereals to wake up our taste buds. Use low to moderate amounts of sugar, salt, white flour, and fats. Revel in new flavors.

SMELL—Even your sense of smell can help you to be healthier. Burn a scented candle. Fill a bowl with potpourri and put it in the living room. Place a fragrant bouquet of flowers on your bedside table. Find a room freshener you like. Use bubble baths and body lotions that make you feel good and smell great. Vanilla, lavender, pine, and cinnamon are some of the most common scents used to produce a sense of well-being.

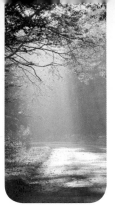

NEED A VACATION?

**Try this twenty-second (or much longer!)
mental vacation**

WANDER THROUGH YOSEMITE NATIONAL PARK, WALK along a white-sand Hawaiian beach, or browse in antique shops in Pennsylvania. By taking time "away" you will resettle or "re-sync" your mind and be able to face your day with new energy.

Come to *www.CREATIONHealth.com* and view a short online video for each letter in the CREATION acronym. Let your mind escape to the scenic environment and take it in as if you were right there. Can you feel the breeze? Smell the freshly cut grass? Hear the encouragement? Then you must be on *CREATIONHealth.com*.

Other helpful things you'll find on the website:

- Take a self-assessment and learn how healthy you really are.
- Learn tips on how to help your kids be healthier.
- Watch an inspirational devotional online video to encourage you.
- Download free CREATION Health wallpapers to stay focused and inspired throughout the day while working at your computer.
- Discover new resources for your healthy lifestyle, including books, videos, seminars, music, conferences, and other resources.

WWW.CREATIONHEALTH.COM

Is it physically harder for you to do the simple things you once did?

Have you wondered why you've lost the energy and stamina you used to have years ago?

Would you like to know how to lower your risk of early death by 20-40 percent?

Do you want to become less susceptible to physical injury?

Would you like to breathe better, sleep more soundly, and lower your chance of getting a headache?

Do you wish you could motivate yourself to get more exercise?

The "A" in CREATION Health stands for Activity.

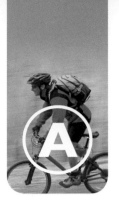

ACTIVITY

CHAPTER 5

The Real Fountain of Youth

ACTIVITY MEANS FINDING EVERY MUSCLE YOU CAN and using it! God made all of those muscles for a reason and designed us so that activity is key to living his prescription for full life. Active people are more alert, energetic, fun, caring, and alive!

Activity strengthens the body to fight disease. In fact, purposeful activity may be the best medicine for fighting almost any disease. It helps the body battle stress, anxiety, and depression. It enables you to sleep better, look better, and feel better. It's all part of God's plan to fill your daily adventure with joy, peace, hope, love, patience, kindness, and good health.

So go ahead and get active. The benefits of a healthier life await you!

SCIENTIFIC SUPPORT FOR ACTIVITY

A recent report by the US Centers for Disease Control summarizes the scientifically proven benefits of physical activity, listed below, then unpacks and documents each claim. The paper, available online, says: "Regular physical activity is one of the most important things you can do for your health. It can help:

- Control your weight
- Reduce your risk of cardiovascular disease
- Reduce your risk for type 2 diabetes and metabolic syndrome
- Reduce your risk of some cancers
- Strengthen your bones and muscles
- Improve your mental health and mood
- Improve your ability to do daily activities and prevent falls, if you're an older adult
- Increase your chances of living longer

"If you're not sure about becoming active or boosting your level of physical activity because you're afraid of getting hurt, the good news is that moderate-intensity aerobic activity, like brisk walking, is generally safe for most people. Start slowly. Cardiac events, such as a heart attack, are rare during physical activity. But the risk does go up when you suddenly become much more active than usual. For example, you can put yourself at risk if you don't usually get much physical activity and then all of a sudden do vigorous-intensity aerobic activity, like shoveling snow. That's why it's important to start slowly and gradually increase your level of activity.

"If you have a chronic health condition such as arthritis, diabetes, or heart disease, talk with your doctor to find out if your condition limits, in any way, your ability to be active. Then, work with your doctor to come up with a physical activity plan that matches your abilities....

"What's important is that you avoid being inactive. Even sixty minutes a week of moderate-intensity aerobic activity is good for you. The bottom line is—the health benefits of physical activity far outweigh the risks of getting hurt.

"Everyone can gain the health benefits of physical activity—age, ethnicity, shape, or size do not matter."[26]

THE REAL FOUNTAIN OF YOUTH

In 1493, Spanish explorer Juan Ponce de León stepped aboard a ship bound for America. He would share the voyage with famed explorer Christopher Columbus, who was on his second journey to the New World. Ponce de León didn't embark on the expedition merely to experience a sightseeing trip, however. He set sail with one goal, one vision, one desire in mind: to find the legendary fountain of youth—that mythical spring of water that would grant eternal youth to the one who drank from it.

De León had many amazing adventures in the New World. History credits him as the first European to discover Florida. Conquering Puerto Rico, he eventually became its governor. But for all his long years of searching, he never discovered what his heart desired most—the source of perpetual youth.

Physical fitness can neither be achieved by wishful thinking nor outright purchase.
— Joseph Pilates

Hundreds of years later, people still continue Ponce de León's quest. Rather than searching for the fountain of youth in some undiscovered land, however, many today seek youthful vitality in pills, therapies, and special diets.

Is there a *real* source of eternal youth in this world? Not that we know of. But many researchers believe they have found the closest resource we have for fulfilling the promises of the legendary fountain of youth. It is simply physical activity.

When physically challenged through regular exercise, the human body grows stronger and healthier, and ages more slowly. In fact, according to the American Heart Association, regular activity has many whole-person health benefits, including great gains for the mind, body, and spirit, and even for social relationships.

Research has shown that with regular physical activity, a person sleeps better.[27] Mentally, an active person handles stress more effectively; he or she is able to think more clearly and generally has a more positive outlook on life.[28] Socially, people often gain more confidence because they feel and look better. And spiritually, those who exercise often find a deeper connection to their Creator, who made them for a life of health, happiness, and peace.

Dear friend, I pray that all goes well for you. I hope you are as strong in body, as I know you are in spirit.
—Apostle John

However, the US Preventive Services Task Force has stated that more than 70 percent of the population in the United States is not physically active.[29] In fact, inactivity is said to be one of the greatest public health challenges of this century. Recent findings suggest that the incidence of stroke and type 2 diabetes would be lower, high blood pressure could be prevented or reduced, and bone fractures would occur less often if Americans just moved more.[30] Many doctors are quick to admit that heart exercise is "Job 1." There aren't any magic bullets in medicine, but the nearest to one is physical activity. People who are physically active cut their risk of heart disease in half.[31]

EDEN'S ACTIVITY

Activity is an important part of the CREATION Health model and a vital component of wholeness. And again, this principle goes right back to the Garden of Eden.

The original paradise was indeed a beautiful, tranquil place. But contrary to some stereotypes, Adam and Eve didn't lie around all day on a riverbank in Eden, drinking fresh coconut milk. They didn't just lounge around looking at flowers and birds. While God could have designed their lives to be quite labor-free and passive, he had something else in mind.

"The Lord God took the man and put him in the Garden of Eden to work it and take care of it" (Gen. 2:15). Paradise, for Adam and Eve, wasn't a world of idleness. Eden didn't automatically meet all their needs. They were responsible for cultivating the garden. Perhaps this was God's way of keeping them physically active.

Studies done by Steven Blair at the Cooper Institute for Aerobics Research and by other groups have revealed the enormous influence of exercise on our daily lives.[32] Simply getting up off the couch and walking for thirty to forty minutes three to five times a week can diminish our risk of premature death from cancer and cardiovascular disease by 20 to 40 percent. If I told you that I could give you a 20 to 40 percent return on an investment, you'd probably write me out a check right now.

"Exercise," explains physical therapist Terry Barter, "is the component that brings in the nutrients via the bloodstream to your muscles, your bones, and your joints. It helps get the oxygen through your blood system. This helps grow, mend, promote, and maintain your body. When you take in your car for a tune-up, it really runs better. Then after a while, it needs another tune-up. The body is the same way. Activity is the way we tune up."

EXERCISE AND THE MIND

Physical exercise affects more than just our bodies. It also helps our minds.

Our bodily organs are intricately interrelated. Everything inside us influences everything else. The state of our lungs determines the condition of our heart. Our stomach affects our intestines. Beyond that, our physical condition can sway our mind. Perhaps you've heard about how our mental outlook or our level of stress can impact our physical health. Well, that's a two-way street. Mind affects body. But body also affects mind. And regular exercise can improve our overall attitude. In fact, exercise has a variety of psychological effects that enhance mental health. It buffers against stress, is an effective treatment for anxiety, and according to some researchers, is as effective as psychotherapy in treating mild depression.[33]

LIFE-CHANGE STORIES

Listen to the stories of two people for whom increased physical activity has made all the difference:

Jim, director of purchasing, age fifty-nine; activity of choice: walking

"One year ago I was feeling pretty sick. Some examinations revealed that I had diabetes. I needed to make some changes in the way I took care of myself, otherwise I would increase the likelihood that I would have further complications.

"I started attending education classes on diabetes that brought me up to speed with what I had to do to change my eating habits. I learned how a good exercise routine and weight loss program could make dramatic improvements in my particular health situation. So I decided to start walking.

"When I began, I had to go pretty slowly, because I couldn't tolerate more than a mile at a time. But through the summer I kept at it, gradually building up stamina. Now I walk five miles every morning before I go into work. I've dropped forty-five pounds off my weight, and during my latest visit with my doctor, he officially took me off medication altogether. The exercise program had kept my blood glucose at the same levels it was when I was on medication. I've been able to get my life and health back under control.

"The best result, I think, is that I feel so much better than I did a year ago. I'm healthier. The walk in the morning takes about one hour and fifteen minutes. It gives me time to reflect and get my mind prepared for the day ahead. In addition to the physical benefits of exercising, it's helped me to organize my thoughts and think things through in a way that I didn't have the time to do before I began walking. If I don't have thoughts that need sorting, it's a wonderful time for quiet meditation.

"I wish you could talk to my wife about the changes in me. She says I'm a totally different person. My attitude is more positive, and I'm less prone to be short-tempered. She's happy that I've gotten this thing under control.

"The best tip I could give you is: *persevere*. Don't give up. You'll need to assume a tremendous amount of discipline to get it done. But while changing life habits takes a lot of work and commitment, it's worth it."

Wendy, office manager, age thirty; activities of choice: walking, running

"I never had to watch my weight until after the birth of my second child. Those ten extra pounds wouldn't go away, and my weight continued going up from there. One day I woke up, looked at myself, and said, 'I can't live like this anymore. I have to do something about it.'

"I started an active exercise program about a year ago as a New Year's resolution. Since then I've lost twenty-four pounds. Actually, I lost the weight in the first six months of training, and for the past six months I've held steady. For a while I tried to lose just a bit more, but I've stopped. My body seems to be telling me this is the right weight for me.

"At first I started out with a simple exercise program, walking regularly, then worked my way up to running. Since then I've participated in two small races—each of them five kilometers. Before I started the program I was drinking six to eight Cokes per day, but I quickly cut those out. Caffeine withdrawal gave me tremendous headaches, and I became grumpy. But that time quickly passed, and I had no further problems. Now I mainly drink water.

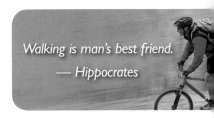

Walking is man's best friend.
— Hippocrates

"Not only do I feel better physically, but I also perform better mentally—partly because I know that I look better. It's nice to hear people say, 'Wow, I didn't even recognize you. You look great!' That gives me more satisfaction than anything, and it really cheers me.

"My routine has affected my family. As soon as I started my weight loss program, my mother did the same thing. She's now dropped about sixty pounds, and it's made such a difference. So my husband decided to get into the spirit. He started exercising with us, and he's taken off thirty-five pounds. It's really nice to do a program with someone else. We can compare weights and encourage each other.

"If someone were to ask my advice about starting an activity program, I would tell them to realize that it is a lifestyle change. I thought there was no way I could lose fifteen pounds. But I tell you, when that first five pounds dropped, I thought, *Wow, this is so great!* Then I had a real goal: if I could lose five, I could go all the way. You don't have to be obsessive about weight loss. Just live a healthy lifestyle and let your body find its natural weight."

ADVICE FROM THREE PROFESSIONALS

Jeannine, Physical Therapist

"When someone comes to a physical therapist for help, we usually focus our efforts on three areas: strength, endurance, and flexibility. These are the three key components of a physically sound body. Many people forget that it is important to focus on improving the condition of the whole body, not just one particular area. We often begin by establishing an exercise program that concentrates on strength training.

"One of the major health problems people face today in our country is inactivity. When people are inactive or have very low levels of activity, their muscles begin to atrophy. That means they get smaller and weaker.

"A hundred years ago people got most of the exercise they needed just by doing their chores and other daily activities. It kept them strong enough that they didn't need health clubs, stationary bikes, or exercise programs to stay healthy. Today, however, with our sedentary lifestyles, we have to make a conscious, consistent effort to exercise and stay healthy so our muscles don't grow small and weak.

"Because our bodies are living, changing organisms, it is really impossible for us to stay at a constant level of health physically, so we must strengthen our body by challenging it, pushing it bit by bit. Some people deceive themselves by thinking that if they just eat healthfully they will have good health. While a good diet is important, it's not enough. If you're not challenging your body, you're not strengthening it, and all the functions of your body start declining.

"Another problem with inactivity is that inactive muscles become stiff and more open to injury. That makes flexibility a crucial part of physical conditioning. When you are active and challenging your muscles, a stretching process takes place that adds flexibility and strength, making injury less likely.

"When I work with patients, I try to emphasize the importance of being active every day, not just two or three times a week. I usually give them 'homework,' exercises they can do at home. As we get closer to the end of our treatments, I encourage them to maintain their exercise in any way that motivates them. As soon as people stop exercising, they start getting weaker again, so it's very important to remain active.

"Endurance, built up by aerobic and cardiovascular training, is also a vital component of physical health. Such exercises work the heart and lungs, causing them to become stronger and more efficient. Endurance exercise elevates the heart rate for a sustained period of time and gives you more energy throughout the day. This type of exercise is especially important for people who spend most of their day on a job that doesn't require much physical exertion. When you train your heart through endurance training, you will have more energy!

Methinks that the moment my legs begin to move, my thoughts begin to flow.
— Henry David Thoreau

"Strength training, flexibility training, and endurance training. Be sure to include all of them in your exercise plan. You will feel less tired, you will feel more motivated, and you will have a greater joy for life in general. Activity makes you feel good!"

Brenda, Registered Nurse and Health Educator

"When a patient first comes into my office and clearly is not living at an optimum level of health, I usually begin by asking them what kind of exercise they get. Unfortunately, the typical answer is 'I do not exercise at all.'

"Many patients I see get so little exercise that they have a hard time just doing day-to-day things. They are in such poor physical shape that just the effort it takes to move around is extremely tiring.

"When I think about the importance of activity, several of the patients I work with come to mind. One of them is a little woman in her seventies who has diabetes type 2, which means she's not on insulin but taking the antidiabetic medication. She was having a difficult time keeping her blood sugar levels in the proper range. I challenged her to start a regular walking program, exercising every day, if possible. She did and brought her blood sugar levels down about thirty points in three months while also losing five or six pounds. When she came back for a follow-up visit she was glowing. Sold on walking, she is determined to make these changes stick for the rest of her life.

"Anyone can exercise. If you are homebound, there are all sorts of interesting exercises that can be done in the home just for the legs. If you can get to a shopping mall, most malls have daily walking programs in which you can stroll with others in safety before the stores open.

"The most difficult part to adopting a more active, healthy lifestyle is not picking what kind of exercise to do, where to do it, or how often to do it. It is actually doing it!

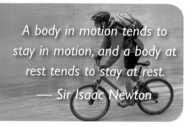

A body in motion tends to stay in motion, and a body at rest tends to stay at rest.
— Sir Isaac Newton

"We urge three helpful tools for our patients:

Find an Exercise Partner. If you have a buddy you have to meet at the corner or who is going to stop by and pick you up, it is a great motivator.

List the Benefits. When you write down the anticipated benefits, you are more likely to stick with an exercise activity. Think about losing weight, breathing better, sleeping more soundly, avoiding headaches, not feeling so fatigued, and finding new joy with your friends and family.

Consider the Alternatives. If you don't exercise, your chances of premature death go up dramatically. In addition, your everyday quality of life goes way down. Why would you want to do that to yourself?

"It's not just adults who are experiencing serious health trouble these days. Recent studies have shown an ever-increasing problem with childhood obesity. Some reports indicate that the number of overweight children is doubling every ten to twenty years. Unfortunately, children learn from adults. They watch us and learn that it is okay to sit in front of a television or computer for hours and hours. Less and less often we see children outside running around the yard, jumping rope, climbing trees, riding bikes, and swimming. But these are normal things children like to do, activities that will help them enjoy God's prescription for health.

"One of the best things for a healthy family to do together is to participate in more physical activities. Plan events that get you into the outdoors doing active things you find enjoyable. Activities shared together are rewarding, both in terms of growing relationships and increased health."

Rhonda, Medical Doctor, Family Practice Physician

"In my primary care practice I've found that there is almost no patient who cannot benefit by increased physical activity. In fact, I believe such activity may be the best medicine there is for practically any health problem because it strengthens the body to fight disease. I think people grasp this principle instinctively because they usually tell me, 'Oh, yeah, I know I need to exercise more.'

"The reason so many don't exercise isn't really a lack of awareness; the problem is busy schedules that lead to overloaded lifestyles. Once we abandon exercise, everything starts to flop out of kilter. Weight goes up, we do not sleep as well, anxiety increases, sugar gets out of control, blood pressure creeps up, and cholesterol rises.

"But none of that needs to happen. Exercise makes a difference! In my experience, people uniformly feel better and sleep better when they exercise. That's 100 percent of the time!

"When active people have fallen out of practice, I remind them about how good they felt and the results they achieved when they were active. If those memories can be restimulated in their brain, they are much more likely to say, 'Yeah, I need to start doing that again, because I felt so much better then.' Some remember how their blood sugar stayed under control or their blood pressure lowered. Others recall how they gained ten pounds in three months when they stopped exercising. If I can reconnect them to the positive things they remember from when they were active, it's much easier for them to get back into it again.

"If people have never been very active, or they tell me they hate exercise, that's much more difficult. I may start by reminding them of some of the benefits they will reap from getting active. We're not discussing the Olympics here—we're talking about starting out just ten minutes a day. Most people tell me that they can do ten minutes a day. Then I ask them if they can do it every day. If not, I get them to do it as many days a week as they can. Ten minutes a day can help you feel 100 percent better!

"Occasionally someone will ask me what my favorite exercises are for staying healthy. That's easy. My favorite exercises are just that—doing whatever I enjoy most.

"Whatever physical activity that you can do and enjoy doing is what you should do. For example, if an older individual tells me that they love to pull weeds in their garden or work in their yard for fifteen minutes at a time, I say, 'Wonderful.' I recommend what is easiest and most economical, because that is what is going to be incorporated with the best success.

"When we talk about exercise, we often discuss it in terms of its benefits to such conditions as diabetes, hypertension, cholesterol, and heart disease. Three of the best results of consistent exercise are stress release, depression release, and insomnia release. Though we don't talk about it much, increased activity can significantly improve all these conditions, because it raises the level of the endorphins in our body that are the body's own 'uppers.' Activity dissipates epinephrine and norepinephrine, the stress hormones. It drops the levels of cortisol, an immune system depressor. A number of studies show that a program of activity over a period of several weeks is as effective as a prescription antidepressant for depression treatment.

"I also believe it is more difficult to listen to what God is whispering into our souls when we are overstimulated. If we can exercise while enjoying nature, it can be a time when we really come together mentally, emotionally, and spiritually. Such activity helps us to calm down, quiet the spirit, and silence the clamor in our brain. Exercise provides time to decide where we're headed and what choices are best. It allows us time to examine what God thinks and what he wants us to do versus what society or our employer is demanding that we do. All of us need to have quiet time to stop and process.

"By the way, exercise can also improve our relationships. Take a revitalizing walk in the evening or a refreshing walk in the morning with someone you love. Couples who do tell me it is one of the best times they have for sharing together. It's an opportunity for coming together, of cherishing each other without a lot of distractions.

"The act of exercising is an antidepressant—encouraging, strengthening, feel-good-about-yourself medication in and of itself. It puts you in a frame of mind to enable you to relate more positively to people around you. No pill can do that as well as muscle movement, especially when it is done outdoors regularly with friends!"

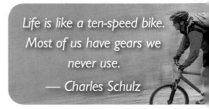

Life is like a ten-speed bike. Most of us have gears we never use.
— Charles Schulz

If you get bored with walking, get creative. Walk to the grocery store and reward yourself with a bottle of juice or the most luscious peach in produce. Listen to books or inspirational messages on audio, or snap in your favorite music and whistle while you walk. To add a different dimension to exercise, try using your walking time to pray for your neighbors as you pass by their homes, as well as for other matters you want to talk with God about.

Whatever our individual tastes and limitations, God has designed us for meaningful activity. It should always be a part of our lives.

SUCCESS STEPS

Here are six practical steps to energize your *ACTIVITY* success:

CHECKUP—Always see your doctor before starting any exercise program. Getting a complete physical exam is a great way to start.

Tell your doctor you want to start exercising more and make a plan to get regular checkups and encouragement from your physician.

PARTNER—If possible, find an exercise companion. You will have more fun and will be more likely to continue your exercise program if you have someone to do it with.

AEROBIC EXERCISE—Aerobic exercise consists of three phases: warm-up, aerobic, and cooldown. The warm-up is designed to gradually increase heart rate and body temperature. Muscles that are warm before vigorous exercise are less likely to be injured. Normal walking and light jogging are great warm-up activities. The aerobic phase elevates the heart rate and breathing, making your heart and lungs stronger. Many activities are aerobic in nature, such as fast walking, jogging, biking, swimming, and aerobic dancing. Ideally, you should work your way up to sixty minutes of activity three times a week. The cooldown allows for a slow, gradual recovery of your heart rate and prevents pooling of blood in your lower extremities. Slow walking is an appropriate cooldown activity. It is important to wear comfortable clothing to allow free movement when exercising. It is also a must to wear appropriate shoes to reduce the possibility of injury and strain on the feet.

STRENGTH TRAINING—Strength training is done to improve the overall strength and endurance of muscles not used during the aerobic phase. Pushups, pull-ups, crunches, and lower and upper body weight lifting are all beneficial. It isn't necessary to have expensive weights to do this. Use a can of vegetables. Take an empty milk jug and add some water. Anything that adds resistance will strengthen your muscles. Don't be tempted to overdo it. Listen to your body and use the appropriate amount of weight. If you can do more than twelve repetitions, the weights may be too light. If it is difficult to do even eight repetitions, the weights are probably too heavy. Gradually build up to heavier weights.

STRETCHING—Stretching is often ignored as part of a balanced exercise program. It promotes maximum flexibility by working muscles and joints through their full range of motion. All major muscles should be stretched, especially those that are used during your workout. It is important to not bounce or jerk while you stretch, which might cause injury to the muscle. Stretching should always be slow and controlled.

EVERYDAY ACTIVITIES—Don't forget other daily activities that will increase movement. Take the stairs instead of an elevator at work whenever possible. Vacuum and mop the floors in your home. Mow the lawn (a riding lawn mower doesn't count). Play actively with children. Ride a bicycle to visit a friend. Jump rope or do pushups during television commercials.

Have you ever been let down by someone you trusted?

Have you ever felt worthless because of another person's opinion of you?

Do you sometimes live in fear of what the future might bring?

Have you ever been angry with God?

Have you ever found yourself struggling to pray?

Do you have a sense of purpose in your life?

The "T" in CREATION Health stands for Trust in Divine Power.

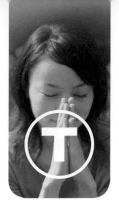

TRUST

CHAPTER 6

How Faith Improves Your Health

GOD ORIGINALLY DESIGNED US TO BE HIS FRIENDS. But often our lives are so busy that we leave little time for him. Those are the times we try to go it alone, without the wisdom and energy his friendship offers. Yet without him, our daily activities can become pointless. We're busy, but we just don't know why.

Trust in God works like a gyroscope. It keeps you stable even if life places you on a precarious angle. The reason that a gyroscope achieves stability is found in its inner mechanism. The same could be said of you or me. If our inner world revolves around trust in God, we remain centered and stable, no matter how our outer world is spinning.

When we trust in God, we are transformed from people of fear to people of courage—and from people of courage to people of purpose.

It's been said that courage is simply fear that has said its prayers. True. When I'm alone in the world, I can feel a little frightened. With God by my side, I have courage to face the future.

SCIENTIFIC SUPPORT FOR TRUST IN DIVINE POWER

A study reported that people who pray to a God they know intimately are happier, more satisfied, and enjoy a deeper sense of well-being about the direction their lives are headed. In addition, those with faith-filled allegiance are significantly less likely to experience physical illness, mental symptoms, or difficulties with keeping strong relationships.[34] Researchers have offered many explanations. These range from adherence to the healthy lifestyle prescribed by religious teachings to divine intervention. Future studies will be required to identify the reason that trust in a divine power is a pathway to optimal physical and mental health. In the meantime, the scientific data suggest that opening your heart to God will enrich you in ways beyond improved spiritual health.

Trust in divine power has the potential to influence many aspects of mental and physical health. Depression, for example, is a condition (or disorder) in which people feel "pressed down" by life. It can be triggered by a major upheaval in your life and can, by itself, cause major changes in your health. Scientists have shown that depression can worsen the symptoms of pain, result in increased reporting of physical illness symptoms, and lessen the likelihood that its victims will engage in healthy pursuits.

Some studies suggest that faith in a personal God may reduce or counteract depression. This is especially true of those with personal and daily contact with a God whom they believe cares about them as a father cares for his child. Further, support from others who believe similarly (such as fellow church members) may also be a key indicator of a healthy emotional life.[35, 36]

In their award-winning book *New Light on Depression*, Drs. David Biebel and Harold Koenig describe six hidden benefits of depression that can only be seen through the lens of faith, including showing us how much we need God. "Depression has a way of permanently etching the words: 'I need God' upon one doorpost of your heart," say the authors. "Before depression is finished with you, on the other doorpost will be etched: 'I need others.' Our struggle with emotional pain demonstrates forever our inability to conquer such forces by ourselves. We need help, both human and divine. Depression does away with our pride and self-sufficiency, taking the ground of our self-reliance and self-confidence out from underneath us. Both of us can attest to having learned this lesson—the hard way."

The authors describe the tendency of those who are depressed to expend a lot of energy trying to recapture the past, energy that is simply wasted. "For God dwells in the eternal present: he invites us to dwell there with him by embracing the now of our lives, as, having resolved things in our past that bind, we walk with him toward a [brighter] future..." [37]

Looking beyond depression, a study of 865 high school seniors revealed that students who go to church are less likely to become delinquents, drink alcohol, or use marijuana than other teens—an observation that applied to both boys and girls.[38] Apparently, in maintaining a healthy society, there is an important role for a strong faith in God as well as having a balanced moral education.

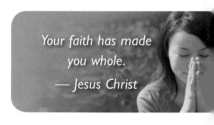

Your faith has made you whole.
— *Jesus Christ*

HOW FAITH AFFECTS YOUR HEALTH

A well-documented report by British Drs. Alex Bunn and David Randall about the health benefits of faith states: "Evidence from over 1,200 studies and 400 reviews has shown an association between faith and a number of positive health benefits, including protection from illness, coping with illness, and faster recovery from it. Of the studies reviewed in the definitive analysis, 81 percent showed benefit and only 4 percent harm. The raw data from some large studies show a significant benefit in mortality for those involved in organised religion. For instance, one study followed 21,204 representative American adults over nine years, and correlated death rates with religious activity and a large range of other data. Income and education had surprisingly little impact, but those who attended church regularly had a life expectancy seven years longer than those who did not. For black people the benefit was fourteen years."

The authors conclude, "In contrast to the popular myth that Christian faith is bad for health, on balance, and despite its limitations, the published research suggests that faith is associated with longer life and a wide range of health benefits. In particular, faith is associated with improved mental health."[39]

Ted Hamilton, MD, author of the books *Building Bridges* and *Wholly Healthy*, states, "I fully believe—and there is research that's beginning to support the notion—that trust in someone outside of yourself actually releases healing hormones into our bodies that contribute to the healing process. Now, the research is not as definitive as we'd like for it to be, but my guess is that five years from now we will view trust and hope as medications to help people recover more quickly."

> *Those who in everything make God first and best, are the happiest people in the world.*
> — E. G. White

The scientific data is growing. Georgetown University Medical School professor Dr. Dale Matthews and his colleagues have shown that religious involvement helps people avoid illness, recover from it more quickly, and most remarkably, live longer. The more spiritually committed you are, the more you benefit.[40] Medical internist Dr. Larry Dossey and others have published rather extensively on the benefits of prayer and healing. Undeniably, the medical community has a growing respect for the role that faith and prayer play in our overall well-being.

"I found that people who are faced with disease," continues Hamilton, "who are also fearful about the ultimate outcome, have more difficulty focusing on recovery. But those who have, beneath all the concerns and worries and challenges of that illness, an underlying trust, a trust that says things will ultimately work out for the good because God loves and cares for them—they're somehow able to marshal resources that contribute to their healing in ways that others aren't able to."

A HEALING FAITH AT THE END OF LIFE

Faith is an essential part of healing as well as a vital aspect of wholeness. It can keep us strong even when we're physically at our weakest. And it can sustain us even when our bodies are losing the battle for life.

Hospital chaplain Jay Perez, author of the book *The Patient Experience* has found this to be true for many of the patients he counsels. "Some people have to face the reality of a terminal illness or a crisis situation," he says, "and where do they turn? At such times faith and trust in God become extremely important, because faith in God gives strength that allows people to cope with such overwhelming news. In fact, sometimes after the death of a loved one, a strong reliance on God may be the only thing that helps people deal with the tragedy. It's the belief that he will take care of us—even after death—that allows people to be able to find the strength to cope."

A GROWING FAITH

As you'll recall, God surrounded Adam and Eve with living things that were very good (see Genesis 1). He wanted them to be fully convinced that he cared enough to provide for all of their needs. He especially wanted them to have a healthy relationship with him. But he didn't want it to stop there. Everything in the Creation story teaches us that faith and trust are grown, not simply given. It's evident that even Adam and Eve had to grow in their confidence in God. As it was then, so it is today—faith is a process, not an on or off switch.

At first they stumbled in their relationship with God. He had warned them about one spot in Eden where they should not go—the tree of the knowledge of good and evil. That's where a deceiver lay in wait. Holding a grudge against God, Satan (as the Bible calls him) desires to destroy God's children any way he can. Eve saw a delightful fruit hanging there. It looked good. *What harm could there be in it?* Eve must have thought. So she listened to the serpent instead of the voice of the Father who loved her and had provided for her. Eve ignored divine instructions and ate the fruit. Then she convinced Adam to share it with her. And just that quickly, both the man and the woman had shattered the relationship of trust God was building in the garden.

But God didn't just leave it alone. He had some choices to make:

Do I leave this planet to die on its own?

Do I destroy this world and start over with a new one?

Do I do something to win my creation back from the consequences of their own choices?

Infinitely wise and loving, God considered one outcome—the redemption of his creation. He went looking for the people he'd made in his own image, the people he had lovingly created. His only thought was to restore their broken relationship with him and rebuild that trust.

In today's world, filled with conflict and upheaval, we humans need to trust in a loving, powerful God, especially when our impulses lead us in a direction that is away from his design, his best intentions. Adam and Eve learned the hard way that trusting a caring Creator is better than trusting their own desires.

Faith is a process. It is something we grow into and develop over time and through trials. Most people think they don't have the kind of faith that produces miracles, that perhaps their faith is rather weak. Well, join the club called the human race. Jesus' twelve closest friends, men who are called his *disciples* ("learners"), had the same concern. They were always encountering obstacles that seemed bigger than their faith.

One day, they went up to him and said, "'Increase our faith.' So the Lord said, 'If you have faith as a mustard seed, you can say to this mulberry tree, "Be pulled up by the roots and be planted in the sea" and it would obey you' " (Luke 17:5–6, NKJV).

A tiny seed of faith is what Jesus was saying. That's all it takes. Why? Because what matters most is, in whom do we place our faith? If we place our trust in an all-powerful God, then ultimate good will happen. Why? Because anything is possible within his plan and will for your life. And it's not because our faith is so big—it's because God has a deity-sized view of time, a perspective of your life unlike anyone else.

The Bible tells us that this same God offered the ultimate gift to the world: his one and only Son. He sent his Son to rescue us from the disaster of sin . . . our sinful nature as well as specific things we do that we know are wrong. In the person of Jesus Christ, God the Father gave everything. He held nothing back—because we were in need, and he had the answer for our need.

The apostle Paul, a man well-acquainted with hardship, talks about this awesome generosity in one of his letters: "He who did not spare his own Son, but gave him up for us all—how will he not also, along with him, graciously give us all things?" (Rom. 8:32).

> *Never be afraid to trust an unknown future to a known God.*
> — *Corrie Ten Boom*

That's the God we can trust. We can have absolute confidence in him in sickness and in health. And we can look to him for healing and wholeness.

A CHANGING FAITH

"Trust changes a person's outlook," observes hospital Chaplain Marti Jones. "If you're a trusting person, you are likely more positive. When you know that God cares for you, you are able to rely on the fact that God is leading, even when you don't understand why bad things happen to you or someone you love.

"One of the ministries that I carry on in the hospital is providing spiritual nurture not only for our patients but also for our staff. We have a ministry called People of the Word—POW. Weekly we study the Bible with individuals who want to come together and explore it. That's how I met Barbara."

Barbara will never forget how studying the Bible helped her find a solid trust in God that helped change her entire life.

"The first time I met Marti," Barbara recalls, "I was at a really low time in my life. My husband of thirty-five years had left me, so naturally I was devastated. Then a few months later my mom—full of good health—died suddenly. She had a massive stroke. I felt as if I had nothing left, so I turned to God.

> Any concern too small to be turned into a prayer is too small to be made into a burden.
> — Corrie Ten Boom

"Because we're human," she acknowledges, "it's hard to trust people. But I found that if we trust God fully and hand him all our cares, he gives us peace that truly is beyond our understanding. He provides us the support and the love that we need to make it on a day-by-day, and sometimes hour-by-hour, basis. When your husband leaves you, you feel kind of worthless. Some people in this circumstance reach out to the bottle or to drugs. Others get on the phone and talk to their friends. But I felt full trust in the Lord, because he'll never leave me— and I knew that. I joined the Bible study that Marti was teaching, and since then I've grown closer to the Lord."

Turning to God at crisis points is definitely not unusual. Most people don't call upon their faith or realize their inner strength until they're really faced with a critical life event, such as a diagnosis of cancer or some other life-threatening illness. So how can faith help you get through the hard times?

Dr. David Biebel, author of the book *If God Is So Good, Why Do I Hurt So Bad?* describes the importance of viewing adversity with the eyes of trust:

> One morning not long after my son, Jonathan, had died, I was called to the scene of a fire where six children and their mother had died. Three of the children had been in the children's choir of the church I was pastoring at that time. After walking among the rubble and viewing the charred remains, my vision of realities was sharpened. The starkly grotesque scene of destruction confronted me with the frailty of temporal life and the true significance of the eternal.
>
> Thankfully, the eternal—the life that emanates from God—is bigger, able to swallow up the temporal—what we usually regard as

"life"—so that *"what is mortal may be swallowed up by life"* (see 2 Cor. 5:4). *In the mind of God, there is only one reality, his reality — whether it is seen from our side and labeled "mortal" or from his side and called "life." At all times, by faith we live and move and have our being in him, who is the source of life. Even when it seems like he is not there, he is with us, so we need not be afraid. Doubt whispers, "He is nowhere." Trust counters, "He is now here!"* [41]

A BEGINNING FAITH

The best part about trust is that we don't have to discover it by ourselves. God is there for the journey, guiding and cheering us along. Since the beginning of Creation, God has found a way to deal with the guilt and shame that comes from being human and living on Planet Earth.

The climax of the story of the Garden of Eden is the restoration of intimacy with God. That's what God cares about the most—restored relationship. Spiritual intimacy. God wants to connect each of us to himself, to the Eternal. That's how we find ultimate peace. It's the only thing that can heal the deepest part of us.

So how do you begin your spiritual journey?

The important thing is to start building on the foundation of whatever faith you already have. This will help get the process started and show you that you may not need to start from scratch. Jesus' assurance is that even with a mustard seed of faith we can begin a long and wonderful journey.

I have discovered three practical steps that will help you develop an attitude of trust in God.

FIRST, COMMUNICATE. Trust grows in an atmosphere of honesty and openness. God has been honest with you. It's time to be honest with him as well. You can do that in prayer, which is nothing more than talking to God and listening with your heart for his answers (see Phil. 4:6–7).

SECOND, LISTEN. Be open to what God reveals about himself in his Word, the Bible. You've got to get to know someone better in order to trust him or her, right? So start spending some regular time in understanding the Bible more and more. I suggest you begin with the Gospels (Matthew, Mark, Luke, and John), the accounts of Christ's life on earth. They will provide you with a close-up picture of God's character and let you know exactly what he's like. So take time to really drink in each scene, each encounter, each bit of teaching (see Heb. 1:1–3).

> *When the core of our being is threatened, we find out that trust is not something you have; trust is something you do moment by moment.*
> — Linda Nordyke Hambleton

THIRD, ASK. Start requesting God's help in specific areas of your life. And keep asking. As you continue, you'll begin to learn more and more from the way he answers. His "no" can be as instructive as his "yes" to your prayers. But always ask. That's how you exercise your faith (see Matt. 7:7–8). We would invite you to talk to one of our chaplains. They are dedicated to bringing you closer to God. They can provide you with a book or Bible lessons that will help you to know God.

Always remember that right now you've got faith at least the size of a mustard seed. So use it. Put it to work—and watch your world change.

SUCCESS STEPS

Here are six practical steps to energize your *TRUST IN DIVINE POWER* success:

TOGETHER TIME—The key to developing a trust relationship with someone is to spend time together. The same is true when you spend time with God. Communion between just the two of you is essential to the trust that will lead to better health.

A QUIET PLACE—Do you have a favorite rocking chair, a secluded bench in the park down the street, or a well-worn pew in your church? That may be the perfect meeting place for you and God. Or for some, it may be in the middle of rush hour with the car windows rolled up, the radio off, and the world on hold. Never miss a chance to create a "quiet place" for you and God to communicate.

SCRIPTURE—We all enjoy getting letters from loved ones and friends. Letters keep us connected to the people who are important in our lives. The Bible is God's letter to us. What better way to know God than to read the Bible. Reading the Bible will show us the true, trusting relationship that God is eager to share with us.

PRAYER—It can happen anywhere, anytime, and does not depend upon your posture or words. Prayer is talk—honest talk, fearless talk, friend to friend.

BOOKS—Take a trip to a Christian bookstore. Wander the aisles and look at everything, especially the books under the "Devotional Reading" sign. Choose three or four of the most interesting and take them to the "reading" chair at the back of the store. Scan a page or two out of each, then select one to buy. We can often see God through the words of other Christians who have devoted their life to a strong fellowship with God.

PEOPLE—Are you acquainted with people who seem close to God? Get to know them. Ask questions. Listen. Follow their lead. They just may know the path!

Do certain people frustrate you?

....

Is there someone in your life with whom
you need to make peace but don't
know how?

....

Can you be honest with someone and
loving at the same time?

....

Do you know how to build people up?

....

Do you sometimes feel socially isolated
from people?

....

Would you stand in line for hours to hug a
complete stranger?

....

The "I" in CREATION Health stands for
Interpersonal Relationships.

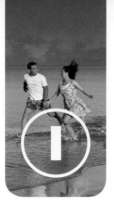

INTERPERSONAL RELATIONSHIPS

CHAPTER 7

Growing Rich through Intimacy with Others

DO YOU VALUE KIND WORDS FROM A CLOSE FRIEND? How about a wholehearted hug in hard times? We encounter many of life's greatest joys while sharing hopes and dreams, hurts and hugs with family and friends. Yet some of these relationships can also be our greatest challenges. People are wonderful—and people are terrible.

That's where God can step in with his box of "relationship tools." The tools God uses with us—such as grace, love, truth, and time—are the same tools we can use with others. These tools are proven to grow, nurture, and even repair relationships. They are designed to help us become healthy humans and compassionate friends.

Relationships are God's number-one priority.

He didn't create this world just so we could have correct information about him (as important as that is). And he didn't send his Son to the earth in the person of Jesus Christ because our behavior was something to be proud of. Just the opposite! The mystery the Bible reveals is that "God is love," and love has no recourse but to give love.

Parents have children because they want to give their overabundance of love away, and God created humans for the same reason. It is his nature to love, and humans created in his image are the recipients of this great and wonderful love.

That's why God is concerned—and has so much to say—about relationships. But as in other areas discussed in this book, God isn't the only one who knows how important relationships are to our overall health and well-being.

SCIENTIFIC SUPPORT FOR INTERPERSONAL RELATIONSHIPS

Did you know that the more friends you have, the less likely you are to catch a cold? That's what Dr. Sheldon Cohen at Carnegie Mellon University has found.[42] Not only that—if you do come down with a cold, the duration and severity of symptoms will be lessened if you have lots of social contacts. Conversely, social isolation is devastating to good health. Friends not only increase your capacity for pleasure; they enhance your ability to heal.

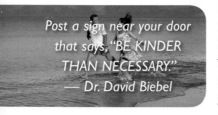

Post a sign near your door that says, "BE KINDER THAN NECESSARY."
— Dr. David Biebel

In a classic study reported in the medical journal *Lancet*, Dr. David Spiegel at Stanford University found that women with breast cancer who participated in psychosocial support groups lived longer than breast cancer patients who did not.[43] Subsequently, investigators at UCLA found that a structured group intervention reduced both mortality and cancer recurrence for the participants.[44]

Sometimes the benefits of a factor are best revealed when examining what happens when it is absent. This is certainly true of social support. Dr. James House reviewed an extensive body of literature that studied a total of 10,000 women. The conclusion was that social isolation increases your risk of dying from all causes. In the Alameda County study, the risk was 2.8 times greater.[45]

GET HEALTHY THROUGH INTIMACY WITH OTHERS

What do block parties and low blood pressure have in common? A small town in Roseto, Pennsylvania, seems to have the answer.

The government discovered that Roseto, Pennsylvania, was one of the healthiest communities in the country. Wanting to find the reason for its superior health when compared to the rest of the country, they sent a group of investigators there. What they discovered was that its inhabitants were very close-knit. If somebody had a difficulty, the community surrounded that person with help. People knew one another, and they would frequently have dinners together. The community's mutual support was way above the norm.[46]

One of the things we're discovering through science is that having a good social support system—deep, personal friendships—can be very beneficial to health. An interesting side note that supports this finding, though in a rather sad way, is that over time, as the habits and makeup of this community have changed, the health status of Roseto now mimics that of the US, overall.

THE HUMAN HEALING INGREDIENT

In his book *Love and Survival*, Dr. Dean Ornish, a physician known for his work in reversing heart disease, speaks about the power of love and intimacy. "I am not aware," he writes, "of any other factor in medicine—not diet, not smoking, not exercise, not stress, not genetics, not drugs, not surgery—that has a greater impact on our quality of life, incidence of illness, and premature death from all causes."

Ornish states that loneliness and isolation increase the likelihood that we may engage in harmful behaviors such as smoking and overeating, that we may get certain diseases or die prematurely, and that we will not fully experience the joy of everyday life. "In short," he observes, "anything that promotes a sense of isolation often leads to illness and suffering. Anything that promotes a sense of love and intimacy, connection and community, is healing." [47] Research from the University of California at Irvine reinforces this point. Its studies indicate that loneliness and lack of emotional support could cause a threefold increase in the odds of being diagnosed with a heart condition. Interestingly, the study also showed that having just one person available for emotional support served to be enough to reduce the risk of heart disease.[48]

ABC News carried the story of a small Indian woman on a worldwide hugging tour. Her name is Mata Amritanandamayi, but some have simply dubbed her the "hugging saint." According to best estimates, Mata has hugged more than twenty million people in countries all across the globe. And she shows no signs of slowing down. On her stops in American cities such as New York, Los Angeles, Chicago, Washington, DC, and Boston, thousands of people line up to be embraced by a complete stranger. When asked where she gets all her energy, she replies simply, "It takes no energy to love. It is easy." Reporter Buck Wolf described his experience with the woman many affectionately call "Amma" or "Mother": "Here I am, in the deep embrace of a stranger. She folds me into her arms, coos into my ear, and gently kisses my temple . . . 'My son, my son, my son, my son,' she says, rocking me back and forth. 'Love you, love you, love you . . .' I look around me. Here are fellow New Yorkers—rich, educated, and hardened to flimflams. Why do these people wait for hours . . . ?

"'I'm not religious,' a twenty-eight-year-old banker tells me. 'I saw her four years ago in Houston. Now, I just go to her every chance I get. She may be just an old woman who hugs. But there is some beauty in this. Maybe we have to appreciate our need to hug and be hugged—to care for each other.'" [49]

People know when they're cared for—when they're loved. And people who are cared for and loved heal more quickly.

A HEART-TO-HEART COMPANION

God knew the value of relationships from the very beginning. He spent six days filling the earth with plants and creatures of all kinds for Adam to enjoy. But that wasn't enough. Though Adam had a garden paradise abounding with an incredible variety of living things, he needed something more. And God knew just what that was. "The Lord God said, 'It is not good for the man to be alone. I will make a helper suitable for him'" (Gen. 2:18).

Living creatures surrounded Adam, but he was still alone deep inside. His soul held a vacuum. He didn't have the companionship of someone like him— another human being. "So the Lord God caused the man to fall into a deep sleep; and while he was sleeping, he took one of the man's ribs and closed up the place with flesh. Then the Lord God made a woman from the rib he had taken out of the man, and he brought her to the man" (verses 21–22).

God used Adam's rib to create the first woman. He could have fashioned her from the dust of the ground, as he did Adam. Or he could have made her from nothing. (That's how God usually worked.) But he took something from Adam's chest, near his heart, to show that this would be a person who would stand by his side. She would be someone who could walk through life with him as a heart-to-heart companion.

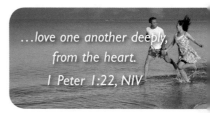

...love one another deeply, from the heart.
1 Peter 1:22, NIV

Adam recognized his soul mate as soon as he set eyes on her. "And Adam said: 'This is now bone of my bones and flesh of my flesh; she shall be called Woman, because she was taken out of Man'" (verse 23, NKJV).

"Bone of my bones, flesh of my flesh"—that's what God created in the Garden of Eden. He brought into being human companionship and intimacy. He knew that close interpersonal relationships were essential for our health and happiness as human beings.

QUALITY IMPROVEMENT

I've discovered that it's not just the quantity of our relationships, but their quality that counts. It's not just how many people we know or how many people we say hi to each day. Rather, it's letting other people really know us. Relationships are most nurturing when we take the time to form that kind of bond.

The quality of our relationships, to a large extent, determines the quality of our lives. The more challenges we face, the more we need other people. One person in a crisis is a tragedy. Two people in a crisis is a support group. A sense of belonging makes people feel cared for, loved, and valued. It provides social comfort and a sense of control throughout life's unexpected twists and turns.

John (not his real name) is a cancer researcher. One day, life threw him an unexpected twist when he was diagnosed with cancer. Upon hearing the news, his family immediately rallied around him and became his support group. "Before I was diagnosed," John said, "when the doctor told me, 'It looks like lymphoma and we need to do some lab tests to find out for sure,' I was in sort of a state of shock. Because here I am working at a cancer institute doing cancer research, and I'm supposed to be safe from this stuff, you know. But it just doesn't work that way.

> *True friends are those who really know you but love you anyway.*
> — *Edna Buchanan*

"When I told my family that my doctor was talking to me about lymphoma, it was difficult, although everybody was very supportive. No one took the attitude that this was the end. Instead, people rallied around me and tried to offer support whenever they could. It is very important for family to be involved in healing. We sometimes don't realize it, but we're greatly affected by the people around us."

When family and friends pull together for the ones they love, something remarkable occurs. Grace happens. Healing takes place. It may not always be a physical healing—it may be just emotional or spiritual. But it's healing, nevertheless.

I think of an unconscious mother in critical care who was not expected to survive. As her children gathered around her, they shared a lot of remorse. "If only I had spent more time with Mom," her youngest son kept saying. "If I just hadn't run away from home . . . I hurt her so badly."

One by one around the group each expressed their regret about things they wished they had said to their mother. As the group prayed together, they asked God to intervene in the situation. Then a miracle occurred. For a short while the mother regained consciousness, and the whole family enjoyed a wonderful time of reconciliation. Everyone said what he or she needed to. The mother brightened up for a considerable period of time then slipped back into unconsciousness. Shortly thereafter she passed away. Yet she did so with a sense of peace and joy that she hadn't known before because all of her relationships were in order. Though the mother did not experience physical healing, her heart and those of her children had emotional healing.

Just as this family found healing in unity, God desires you and me to experience unity with those around us. He wants us not only to be reconciled to him, but also to one another.

DEALING WITH A PAINFUL PAST

Herdley Paolini, PhD, a noted psychologist and author of *Inside the Mind of a Physician*, specializes in helping doctors navigate through difficult life circumstances. Dr. Paolini points out that, when it comes to interpersonal relationships, "Some of us may have experienced deep wounds in our previous relationships. Out of the pain, we may have withdrawn and as a result continue to experience the past pain as well as the loneliness of the present.

"A great deal of our personal growth as well as most of our personal pain are the result of interpersonal relationships. Ultimately then, even though things get broken in relationships, they can also only be healed in relationships.

"Dr. Mark's story illustrates this well. He had experienced a painful divorce where he fought for and lost custody of his two young children. He vowed to himself to 'never' make a commitment to another relationship again. The anger, bitterness, and resentment was at the forefront of every encounter with females—fellow physicians, nurses, girlfriends, and even with males. His one experience with his ex-wife templated his view of others and relationships in general. And yet, he was not aware of how his internal pain was being expressed and how it was shaping his present relationships. It was not until a nurse, tired of being treated poorly, kindly shared with him how she experienced him. Out of that reality check, he luckily searched for professional help. There, he was helped to heal the past pain, enter a process of forgiveness toward himself and the other, learn and grow from the experience, and eventually be able to open his heart to others again. His renewed ability to embrace himself and relationships facilitated a better relationship with his ex-wife and his children and led to a new romantic relationship which ended up in a mutually fulfilling marriage." [50]

If you struggle with difficult relationships from your past, why not do yourself (and those around you) a favor. Don't live in bitterness. Seek professional help or the sympathetic ear of someone who knows and loves you. Dealing with pain from past hurts in a way that helps you heal and acquire skills to develop healthy, safe, and mutually fulfilling relationships, is one of the most important steps we can take toward our overall health.

INVEST IN OTHERS

The basic picture of a healthy relationship that comes to us out of Eden is that of two people clinging together, two people giving themselves to each other.

In a world full of self-absorbed people, it's easy to develop our own little self-contained universes: *my* personal space, *my* boundaries, *my* needs, *my* limits. Technology and affluence—especially in highly developed countries—have made us not nearly as dependent on others as we used to be. Sometimes, of course, this can be a good thing. After all, no one wants to be a burden on someone they love. But we are also more isolated and self-contained. The worst part is that because we invest less in the relationships that really count, we find ourselves emptier.

God knew that we needed to be understood on the deepest level. That's why he performed the first marriage in the Garden of Eden. He joined Adam and Eve together to become one flesh. God designed them to cleave together, to cling to each other.

Our marriages need that kind of commitment today, and our friendships also need a greater measure of intimacy. We find healing and nurture only when we invest time and energy—when we invest ourselves—in other people. Meaningful relationships can develop only when we open ourselves up to others. The truth is, only to the degree that we become honest and transparent before them will we find nurture and healing.

> *A fundamental principle for dealing with hardship is, "We're all in this together."*
> — *Sandy Shugart, PhD*

Adam and Eve knew this kind of transparency. The Bible says, "And they were both naked, the man and his wife, and were not ashamed" (Gen. 2:25, NKJV). Such nakedness is much more than two people without clothing. It is two people who are vulnerable before each other, who have nothing to hide.

That's the kind of relationship God established in the garden. In the beginning he made possible a healthy, honest, accepting companionship. And that's still his plan for each one of us today.

Healthy relationships are gifts that keep on giving, producing healing and wholeness for years to come. You can become a giver today.

SUCCESS STEPS

Here are six steps to energize your *INTERPERSONAL RELATIONSHIP* success:

FAMILY—Learn about your family history and prepare a photo storybook of your heritage. Enjoy a family night once a week or once a month when everyone gets together for dinner or something else fun. Best of all, spend personal time with each family member this week.

FRIENDS—Nurture quality friendships. Step outside of your comfort zone and dedicate special time for others. This will usually revolve around food, walks, games, or sports, with the end result being conversations about everything!

NEIGHBORS—Be attentive and friendly to those who live near you. If you have elderly neighbors, offer to chauffeur them to the grocery store. Welcome new families with pies, breads, or flowers. Offer to mow and edge your neighbors' lawns while they are on vacation.

ORGANIZATIONS—Join a local organization in which you can share your skills and develop new friendships. Become a Big Brother or Big Sister. Help build a Habitat for Humanity home. Read to kids at the library. If you are qualified, coach soccer or Little League.

CHURCH—A church family can easily become the core of your personal support system. Do more than attend; choose to become involved with a service ministry offered at your church that fits where your heart and skills are. Helping others is one of the best ways to boost your health.

WORK—Don't neglect the valuable relationships with your coworkers. Learn about them, their families, and their hopes. In the process, your work may even become easier!

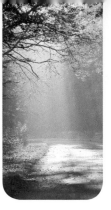

ARE YOU INTERESTED IN BECOMING A CERTIFIED CREATION HEALTH LEADER?

CREATION Health Institute is your place for online training. Our virtual offerings provide a self-paced learning experience as you acquire the skills to become a confident seminar leader.

SEMINARS are a proven way to help people in your business, church, or community become acquainted with the fundamentals of whole-person health. The tools and resources to become a health seminar leader can be found at: CREATIONHealth.com in the "CREATION Health Institute" section. Courses are offered for leaders and students of CREATION Healthy living, including:

- Certification as a CREATION Health Seminar Training Leader
- Lifestyle Training for individual students

WWW.CREATIONHEALTH.COM

Are you constantly fighting
negative thoughts?

....

Have you ever felt helpless to change the
situation you're in?

....

Do you wish you were more positive with
other people?

....

Have you become the negative parent you
vowed you'd never be?

....

Do you become depressed when things
don't turn out as you had hoped?

....

Would you like to know three sure-fire
steps to creating a positive outlook?

....

The "O" in CREATION Health stands
for Outlook.

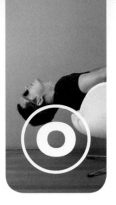

OUTLOOK

CHAPTER 8

Your Mind Can Heal Your Body

OUTLOOK IS A GIFT YOU GIVE YOURSELF, THE COLORS with which you paint the world. Some of us leave smudges of gray and dark purple as we frown through the day. That's our choice. Others leave sparkling designs of gold, green, and sky blue. That's also our decision.

God designed each of us to be different, special, unique, and wonderful. But having a negative outlook is not in his plan. A negative outlook switches off the lights of hope. It changes love to hate, and peace to stress.

A positive outlook does just the opposite. It turns on the lights, ignites love, and allows our heart to focus on possibilities, not problems. He made us to be positive, and his example sets the standard. What could have been more discouraging than to create something as wonderful as the universe, the world, the Garden of Eden, and then watch as the most special and beloved creation—humans—turned against you? Yet God didn't become depressed and mope around heaven for a few thousand years; he went straight to work, making our relationship with him right. Knowing how fallible men and women were, he really must be an optimist!

SCIENTIFIC SUPPORT FOR OUTLOOK

Attitude is more than simply a state of mind. It can influence how the brain manages the healing process. Dr. Richard Davidson at the University of Wisconsin has discovered that people who have a positive attitude have more electrical and metabolic activity on the left side of the brain's prefrontal lobe. This is the side of the brain that, when activated, is associated with greater numbers of natural killer cells—the cells that help us fight viruses and perhaps even cancer. It's not clear which is the chicken and which is the egg, but some studies suggest that simply by thinking positive thoughts you can turn on the side of the brain linked with improved immunity.[51]

Dr. Margaret Kemeny has found that personal expectations are a significant predictor of HIV progression, especially when the person with a pessimistic outlook has experienced loss. The patients in the study had a greater decrease in CD4 T-cells and an elevated increase in serum and cell surface activation markers. Exactly how attitude can influence the prognosis of a patient with HIV is not completely clear. It may somehow trigger changes in the immune system through fear centers in the brain. Or perhaps the negative effect causes the person to give up and ignore options that might improve their health.[52]

IT'S ALL IN YOUR HEAD

We've all heard the phrase "It's all in your head." But new scientific research may be proving that this saying is truer than we ever imagined. The evidence points to a very real correlation between the mind and the body.

In a *Time* magazine article entitled "How Your Mind Can Heal Your Body" Michael D. Lemonick wrote, "More and more doctors—and patients—recognize that mental states and physical well-being are intimately connected. An unhealthy body can lead to an unhealthy mind, and an illness of the mind can trigger or worsen diseases in the body. Fixing a problem in one place, moreover, can often help the other."[53]

Depression is proving to be particularly destructive to physical health. "Depression jumps out as an independent risk factor for heart disease," reports Dwight Evans, professor of psychiatry, medicine, and neuroscience at the University of Pennsylvania. "It may be as bad as cholesterol." [54]

Heart disease isn't the only illness worsened by depression. Those who suffer from cancer, diabetes, epilepsy, and osteoporosis all appear to ". . . run a higher risk of disability or premature death when they are clinically depressed." [55] In fact, 10 percent of diabetic men and 20 percent of diabetic women also suffer from depression—a rate double that of the general population. Depressed diabetic patients are far more likely to have complications, including heart disease, nerve damage, and blindness.[56]

According to studies by Philip Gold and Giovanni Cizza at the National Institute of Mental Health, depressed premenopausal women exhibit a much higher rate of bone loss than those who aren't depressed.[57] An estimated 350,000 women get osteoporosis each year because of depression, according to the *Time* article by Lemonick.[58] Various studies have tied depression to several other diseases, including cancer, Parkinson's disease, epilepsy, stroke, and Alzheimer's.

> *Stress is an expression of fear. Fear and faith are exact opposites and you cannot operate in both at the same time.*
> — *Freeda Bowers*

(It should be noted that some depression is chemical based, caused by a bad mixture of drugs from a person's past, from genetics, or from long-term unresolved distress. Chemically caused depression can often be treated through medical intervention, with the greatest improvement coming through a combination of the right medication at the right dose, and some sort of "talk therapy." While no one "chooses" depression, many choices of outlook can affect those who are depressed, including many who have been diagnosed as clinically depressed.)

Just as depression can paralyze our outlook, so can negative emotions such as anger and fear. A fascinating Duke University study called

"Anger Kills" examined the profile of physicians in medical school to determine their anger scale. (In this case, anger wasn't simply being upset at a particular incident—that can happen to anyone. Anger here meant a life orientation, the explosive personality that routinely resents every small obstacle or irritant. Those physicians high in the anger scale had a greater incidence of heart disease twenty-five years later.) [59]

Following the terrorist attacks on the World Trade Center in New York City, Jonathan Steinberg, chief of cardiology at New York's St. Luke's–Roosevelt Hospital Center, led a study on the city's heart patients. He found that they suffered twice the usual rate of life-threatening heart arrhythmias in the months following the attacks. "Prolonged stress has physiological consequences," Steinberg observed. "These patients experienced potentially fatal events, even though many of them had trouble identifying themselves as unduly fearful." [60]

"The psychological state of fear affects us biologically," said Los Angeles psychiatrist Dr. Carole Lieberman. "People who are anxious drink and eat more. They have more accidents. They're more likely to get colds or suffer heart attacks." [61]

"Stress," adds Afton Hassett, an expert in psychosomatic illness, "almost always comes out in a bodily symptom." [62]

FROM HELPLESSNESS TO OPTIMISM

Several years ago, researcher Martin Seligman performed experiments showing that dogs could be taught to become helpless in various situations. Seligman then applied those same experiments to human beings. He discovered that during the course of our lives we all develop something called "learned helplessness."

How do we change this? Seligman found that through "learned optimism" we can change our outlook so that we begin to believe that we do have a role in altering our lives. While we can't change other people and some circumstances, we can take control of our own lives and take small steps toward transforming our outlook, and in turn, our health and wellness.[63]   Earlier in this book, I cited Holocaust survivor Viktor Frankl's book *Man's Search for Meaning*. Frankl wrote it after spending two years in a Nazi concentration camp. During that time he concluded: "I have very little liberty from a physical standpoint." But, he said, "I have all the freedom in the world to intellectually frame the experiences that come into my life. . . . We who lived in concentration camps can remember the men who walked through the huts comforting others, giving away their last piece of bread. They may have been few in number, but they offer sufficient proof that everything can be taken from a man but one thing: the last of human freedoms—to choose one's attitude in any given circumstances, to choose one's own way." [64]

Dr. David Biebel, co-author of the book, *52 Ways to Feel Great Today*, has every reason to embrace a bleak outlook on life, after losing one son and almost losing another to a genetic disease. In the book's chapter entitled "Be The Bear," he writes about visiting a friend's home and noticing a famous photograph hanging over the fireplace. The photo showed a grizzly bear waiting at the top of a waterfall, mouth gaping, ready to nab a salmon in 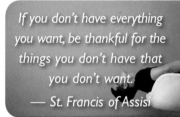 mid-jump. The salmon had been struggling hard to get up over the falls. On one level, the picture seemed bleak. Dr. Biebel remembers identifying with the plight of the poor salmon. *Yup*, he thought, *that's the way life is. Futility. You overcome multiple obstacles on the journey, but then, just when the goal is in sight, the grim reaper points to YOU.*

Dr. Biebel turned to his friend and asked which he identified with most—the bear or the salmon. The friend replied, "The bear." This answer caused the author to reconsider the image, not from the "victim" mentality of the salmon, but from the "victor" mentality of the bear. The more he pondered the implications, the more he liked it. He obtained a poster of the same image. Above the bear and the salmon, in indelible black marker, he wrote "BTB." The letters stand for "Be the Bear." The photo now hangs in his living room.[65]

If you don't have everything you want, be thankful for the things you don't have that you don't want.
— *St. Francis of Assisi*

No one has to be the victim; anyone can be the bear. It's a matter of how you choose to look at things. You do have a choice! Outlook is not the consequence of what others do to you—you are in control of your outlook. So you can opt to see the good. You can choose to see the beautiful, to appreciate what surrounds you. Your choices alter the way you view life, either improving or distorting your perspective.

IN THE JUNGLE, THE QUIET JUNGLE

Believe it or not, these remarkable mind-body discoveries have their roots in the Creation story. This part of the story, though, often gets passed over.

Genesis 2:19 describes what happened after God created the animals. "Out of the ground the Lord God formed every beast of the field and every bird of the air, and brought them to Adam" (NKJV).

Try to imagine the scene. Although Adam was a fully developed man, he was also a newborn in a very real sense. Gazing at all those powerful beasts could have greatly intimidated him. After all, they must have been some pretty fearsome-looking creatures. But notice what God did. "[He] brought them to Adam to see what he would call them. And whatever Adam called each living creature, that was its name. So Adam gave names to all cattle, to the birds of the air, and to every beast of the field" (verses 19–20, NKJV).

Isn't this a wonderful touch in the story of Creation? Why do you think God included Adam in naming the animals? While the Genesis story doesn't give us the reason, I believe God may have included Adam as a way of saying, "Don't be afraid. These are your pets. Give them each a name. They're your playmates." Adam had an entire zoo to play with, a boundless supply of furry and not-so-furry friends.

From the very beginning God sought to instill in Adam a positive outlook on the world around him. He didn't see dangers or enemies—he saw playmates.

A little earlier, the biblical narrative declared that "the Lord God planted a garden eastward in Eden, and there He put the man whom

He had formed" (verse 8, NKJV). God placed him in what he called a garden—a beautiful and magnificent one. He helped Adam view the world as a garden where it was safe to play and safe to grow. He guided him to regard nature as a source of nurture.

In the Garden of Eden, the first human being received a wonderful threefold message:

Play with all your heart.

Live with all your life.

Love with all your being.

It was a positive outlook, a perspective that expects good things. This is another key element in the Genesis story of Creation. And now twenty-first century research affirms this same principle—our outlook, the way we think about life, can help shape our inner world. We have to own our viewpoint, take responsibility for it. Each of us can change our environment from a jungle into a garden—we can turn beasts into playmates.

THINK POSITIVE

Later in the Creation story, God gives us hints for maintaining a positive outlook. His instructions come in the form of a warning to Adam and Eve about the tree of knowledge of good and evil. Notice how he presents it: "And the Lord God commanded the man, saying, 'Of every tree of the garden you may freely eat; but of the tree of the knowledge of good and evil you shall not eat' " (verses 16–17, NKJV).

Fruit trees of every sort filled the Garden of Eden. And God said, "All this is yours to enjoy. There's just one tree—one kind of fruit—that's not good for you."

> *The older you get, the more you realize that kindness is synonymous with happiness.*
> — *Lionel Barrymore*

What's the picture God is reinforcing here? What's the perspective? "Look at all that is good," he is saying. "Keep that in mind. Don't get stuck staring at the bad."

In the New Testament, a man named Paul expands on that positive perspective. "And we know that all things work together for good to those who love God," he tells us, "to those who are the called according to His purpose" (Rom. 8:28, NKJV).

In other words, bad things may happen to us, as Jesus himself said, "In the world you will have tribulation" (John 16:33, NKJV). But God is busy bringing out good in everything. So we shouldn't get stuck in anxiety—we should live in hope.

The opposite of hope is despair or depression. A fifteen-year study done by Kaiser Permanente, the largest managed healthcare organization in the United States, concluded that depressed people utilize healthcare services five times more than the normal population. Thus, teaching people hopefulness may be a way to improve their health.

Dr. Rebecca Moroose, a cancer institute medical director, puts it this way: "People who have hope, people who have a goal, people who have a destiny that they want to see fulfilled, will often live longer than those who curl up and die when they have a serious diagnosis."

In places such as physical therapy clinics, up to 80 percent of recovery relates to mental outlook. As one therapist puts it: "Somebody who has suffered an injury and is needing to physically recover—we've got to see the mental part join in. Getting them inspired—it's a lot of work, it's hard, it's difficult. But to see the daily gains that they can make, this is what's going to inspire them mentally to say, 'You know what, I can do this.'"

I've had the benefit of a father who was very optimistic. In fact, he used to say to me that "discouragement is the devil's anesthesia when he wants to take your heart out." I believe that hope, on the other hand, is the generic drug of the soul.

FORGIVE YOUR HECKLERS

In many cases, choosing hope has a lot to do with letting the past be the past. In the beginning, back in the garden, God modeled an attitude of forgiveness. After all, he'd been wronged. Adam and Eve had eaten the forbidden fruit. They had discounted God's counsel and betrayed his trust in them.

How did God react? Did he turn his back on those who disappointed him? Did he start plotting against them?

No. He didn't hold a grudge or grow bitter. Instead, he showed Adam and Eve how they could find forgiveness.

That's the second essential component of a positive outlook—forgiveness. You have to be willing to forgive others—to let go of the wrongs done to you. If you don't, you will mostly be hurting yourself.

It's been said that bitterness is like taking poison and hoping the other person dies. There's truth to that adage. Holding on to anger is both unproductive and self-destructive. Psychologist Loran Toussaint and his colleagues at the Institute for Social Research at the University of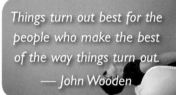

Things turn out best for the people who make the best of the way things turn out.
— John Wooden

Michigan found that forgiving others had a strong link with better self-reported mental and physical health.[66] Other studies have shown that holding on to hostility and the resulting stress this produces can weaken the immune system and increase the risk for heart attack. On the other hand, possessing a spirit of forgiveness can reduce the same risk.[67]

Sports psychologist Herndon Harding tells the story of a baseball player in the Los Angeles Dodgers' minor league system. When something went wrong with his game, the athlete would throw bats or verbally lash out—apparently as a way of preventing other people from criticizing him first. Such behavior, though, made him somewhat of a target, particularly to two fans, who heckled him on a routine and rigorous basis.

Once, after the batter had struck out, the two young men again began taunting him. With a look of determination, the player strode over to the fence where they sat a couple of rows back and gestured to them to come down. The hecklers weren't so sure they wanted to meet an irate athlete carrying a baseball bat, but they gathered their courage and went. Instead of being furious, which would have been his typical reaction, the baseball player now chose to respond differently. Flipping his bat over, he grabbed it by the barrel, extended the handle to the two men, and said, "Do you guys want a Dodgers bat?"

The greatest part of our happiness or misery depends on our disposition and not our circumstances.

— Martha Washington

After that, they never badgered him again. Attending almost every game, they did nothing but support and encourage him just as loudly as they had previously heckled. It was an event that changed the baseball player's life, because he realized that he could choose to react differently. Not only did this alter his outlook; benevolent action actually transformed his environment as well.

He may or may not have known it, but this baseball player followed Paul's advice in dealing with difficult people who've wronged us. "And be kind to one another, tenderhearted, forgiving one another, even as God in Christ forgave you" (Eph. 4:32, NKJV). You see, if we hold on to grudges and hurts, then our hearts sicken, our souls shrivel, and eventually our bodies will physically suffer as well.

SEEING THROUGH GOD'S EYES

Too often when bad things happen to us and we're in pain, we want to blame someone or make someone else hurt. What we need to do is to look for a solution. Instead of projecting our problems onto other people, we need to deal with them. We must stop the blame game and start taking responsibility for our own emotions and behavior.

In the famous "Sermon on the Mount" (see Matthew 5–7), Jesus commented about people with a compulsion to criticize others: "First remove the plank from your own eye, and then you will see clearly to remove the speck from your brother's eye" (Matt. 7:5, NKJV).

Take the plank out of your own eye. In other words, work on your own issues. Don't blame other people—search for a solution that would be healing rather than hurtful. There are three components to a healthy perspective:

First, look for the good.

Second, learn to forgive.

And finally, take responsibility.

It's not just what happens to us; it's how we look at what happens that counts the most. Our perspective determines our progress—in all kinds of life situations.

The story of Donna, a quadriplegic patient, dramatically illustrates this point.

"When I first realized that I was paralyzed and I was going to be in a wheelchair," she remembers, "I was real upset and hurt and felt like somebody owed me—you know, this wasn't fair, why me? Then I realized as time went on that it wasn't going to get much better, so I just needed to accept it. No one was going to beg me to do stuff, so I needed to be the person to continue on with my life and make something, be happy, 'cause, you know . . . it's the best that it's going to be."

"Donna had been in a wheelchair for eleven years before she came to see me," Jeannine, her physical therapist, remembers. "What really impressed me about her was her outlook on life. Although she was still wheelchair-dependent, Donna learned to dress and bathe herself. She made her own food and learned to drive her own car. In fact, she has actually gone back to her profession as a model."

"I didn't think that I'd ever be able to meet a great guy," Donna admits. "But I did and got married. Now I go out and talk to newly injured people and encourage them. Look at me, I tell them. I'm doing fine. Things *will* be okay. You *can* go on."

"After being in a wheelchair for eleven years, it would have been very easy for Donna to have become discouraged, depressed, and maybe even hateful about life," Jeannine observes. "But instead, Donna has taken her situation and become an inspiration to me and to many other people."

"Life is so fragile," Donna says, "and I so appreciate what I have now. And you know, life is not really so bad—it's pretty good. I can still have fun and do things."

A positive outlook can make the difference between progress or paralysis. And God has given us wonderful promises and assurances that can keep us going, even in the worst of times. Here again are three practical tips for improving your outlook.

First, look for the good in situations and in people. You don't have to change your name to Pollyanna to do this, either. It's not that you don't see or accept the bad, but you choose to focus the majority of your thoughts toward goodness.

Second, learn to forgive—don't dwell on the past. Most people want to get things to "even" before they will forgive. The truth is, most offenses against us cannot be made right. That's why giving the gift of forgiveness is often the best choice you can make. In the book *Forgive to Live*, author Dr. Dick Tibbits describes how we are renting space in our head to all manner of painful emotions when we do not forgive. Forgiveness is not admitting someone else is right; it is letting go of being their judge and jury, giving that job to God.[68]

Finally, assume responsibility for your actions, behavior, and emotions. "Own your stuff" is a popular therapist challenge, and it's good advice. When Jesus said, "The truth will set you free," the principle applies to accepting the truth about your own behavior. Do an internal inventory. What kind of attitude have you been carrying with you? Or what attitude do you bring home at night? Take a hard look at your point of view. Does it need some basic adjustments? Could you deal with your problems in a very different way?

SUCCESS STEPS

Here are four practical steps to energize your *OUTLOOK* success:

SELF-TALK—How you talk to yourself plays a major part in whether your outlook is positive or negative. If you are telling yourself that you're a valuable person and a success, you will likely become what you hear yourself saying.

SHIFT ATTENTION—Simply think about something else. Recall happy memories from years gone by, your favorite vacation spots, that person who always was your biggest cheerleader. You'll find that while you visualize the positive experiences, you cannot hear the negative thoughts that were attacking you before. Also, you'll be able to plan what to do next with better perspective and the benefits of an elevated mood.

PUT PROBLEMS ON HOLD—When negative thoughts chase each other through your mind, make yourself an appointment to mull them over later, when you are rested, calmed, and clear-headed. Often things look better away from the spotlight of a low moment, and your responses will be wiser.

WRITE A LETTER—When you're feeling frustrated, write down your negative thoughts as a letter. It might be a letter addressed to a person or a problem. When you write down your negative thoughts, they tend to lose their hold on you. Of course, you never want to send a letter written in anger without waiting a few days. Harry Truman would put such letters in a drawer and leave for a walk. If after a walk he felt as strongly, he'd send it. If not, the letter got edited or thrown away. And never stick that anger in an e-mail and hit send before you have time to really think it over.

Are you confused about what types of diets are best for optimum health?

Do you know what foods you should minimize and maximize at each meal?

Have you fought and lost the "battle of the bulge" too often?

Do you know if carbohydrates are good or bad?

When it comes to animal products, should you use them or not?

Are you ready to make a healthy change in your diet and don't know where to start?

The "N" in CREATION Health stands for Nutrition.

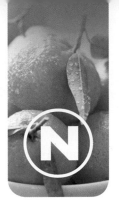

NUTRITION

CHAPTER 9

Eating for Maximum Energy and Healing

GOD DESIGNED US TO GET PEAK PERFORMANCE from the best foods. Then he planted a garden full of them and said, "Enjoy!" We've been reveling in his culinary delights ever since.

When he gave us great food, he also gave us guidelines for enjoying his goodies. Some foods provide the bursts of energy we need in the morning. Others help us slow down in the evening. Certain ones are great in small quantities and terrible by the plateful. Some bring out flavors, while others mask them. The options are many, but the aim is the same. Good nutrition is the process of balancing God's great gifts for full health.

He is the best chef.

SCIENTIFIC SUPPORT FOR NUTRITION

You are what you eat, and that includes your mental well-being. Researchers at Harvard University have discovered that you can adjust serotonin, a brain chemical linked with depression, by varying the amount of carbohydrates in your diet. Not only that, when you get depressed, the brain triggers a craving for the carbohydrates capable of restoring the serotonin to normal. In other words, food can affect your mood, and your mood can influence which foods you choose.[69]

Of all the nutritional options available, one is guaranteed to improve your health and enable you to live longer—eat less. Dr. Robert Good, of the University of South Florida, has conducted research that shows faster regeneration of liver tissue in rats with lower caloric intake.[70] Evidently, illnesses stemming from an unbalanced immune system become easier to manage when calorie intake is limited. No one is certain of why this happens, although the most likely explanation may involve a reduction in lifetime exposure to free radicals (the supercharged atoms that can cause cellular damage and are thought to leave cells at risk for cancer and other diseases) and an increased desire to exercise. Whenever you reach a point during a meal when you'd like more, push the plate away and wait a few minutes instead of automatically reaching for second or third helpings. If you give your body time to digest, the hunger usually subsides, and you'll be exactly where you need to be for optimal health.

By eating the right foods, you might be able to lessen your susceptibility to stress. Ultramarathoners are significantly more vulnerable to upper respiratory infection compared with moderate exercisers. Studies have revealed that when marathoners ingest 5 to 6 percent liquid carbohydrate, it reduces the stress-induced rise in cortisol.[71] The same procedure blocks some of the immune system changes normally associated with excessive exercise. The natural antioxidants in whole foods have also been shown to counteract exercise-induced oxidative stress.[72] While more research is needed, significant progress has been made in this area of study of special interest to elite athletes as well as weekend warriors.

ENRICH YOUR EATING EXPERIENCE

Imagine being able to add healthy, quality-filled years to your life. Consider all the smiles you could share, the new friends you could make, the many lives you could touch. Added years would mean increased opportunities for your own life. Sound too good to be true? It doesn't have to be.

Did you know that the surgeon general's report on nutrition stated that eight out of the ten leading causes of death in the United States have a nutritional or alcohol-related component? And science is constantly confirming this. Research now finds that eating certain foods—fruits and vegetables, whole grains, and plant proteins—can add quality years to your life. Research has shown that a well-balanced diet featuring natural foods is *never* a detriment to human health . . . and many meat-heavy diets can cause a variety of negative health-related issues.[73]

You should know that the advice given in the rest of this chapter will tip very strongly toward the non-meat-eating lifestyle. I realize, however, that many have developed a strong habit and taste for meats in a broad variety. And if it's done in a balanced way, with intake

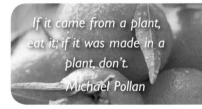

If it came from a plant, eat it; if it was made in a plant, don't.
—Michael Pollan

that includes a lot of fish and poultry, health risks can be lowered. So don't take what is written below as a mandate that a non-meat diet is the only way to live, but rather, eating more natural foods and less meat—especially red meat—should be given serious consideration in order to enjoy optimum health.

Some time ago, an article in *Time* magazine asked, "Should We All Be Vegetarians?" Since then, a number of studies have shown that consuming more plant foods reduces the risk of obesity as well as many chronic illnesses, including heart disease, diabetes, and many cancers, and is likely a factor for a longer, fuller life. More recently, scientific analysis of the "vegan" lifestyle continues, showing similar results.[74]

Research presented at the International Congress on Vegetarian Nutrition indicates that plant-based eating has many healthy benefits. Individuals with diabetes may have fewer complications when consuming more plant foods as well as find it easier to lose weight.

Seniors who choose plant-based eating have a lower death rate and use less medication than those who consume more animal foods. And a plant-based diet increases the intake of heart-healthy fats while lowering saturated fats and cholesterol.[75]

Moderation, balance, and awareness are the key ingredients when choosing plant-based meals. A variety of fruits and vegetables, whole grains, and plant proteins, coupled with the reduction of animal foods, will increase longevity and decrease the risk for most chronic diseases, all factors considered.

George Guthrie, MD, a family physician and Certified Diabetes Educator comments, "I find it rewarding to have patients with type 2 diabetes who are willing to make the change to a diet high in unrefined plant foods. If their pancreatic function is still strong they may actually be able to come off insulin when exercise, fiber, and the antioxidant wonder nutrients of plants are optimized. It's fun to see the smiles, the renewed energy, and the returning zest for living that follows as their blood sugars normalize and the weight comes off."

GOD'S MEAL PLAN

Because God loves us and wants only the best for us, he gave us guidelines for healthy eating. In the Garden of Eden, God created an environment in which Adam and Eve could flourish. It was a fascinating, healthy place filled with plants of every description. God blessed the first human couple and established them as stewards of the riches of Creation. To enable them to fulfill their role, he provided them with healthy food that would sustain them for their work. "Then God said, 'I give you every seed-bearing plant on the face of the whole earth and every tree that has fruit with seed in it. They will be yours for food'" (Gen. 1:29). What did God offer Adam and Eve? A myriad of fruits and vegetables and a wonderful variety of nuts and grains.

But one food God left conspicuously absent in his healthy-eating plan was animal protein. For many years, nutritionists believed that meat, poultry, and fish were the essential sources of protein. They assumed that we must have animal-based protein to have healthy bodies.

However, recent studies show that plant protein not only stacks up well against its animal counterparts, but it also provides other healthy benefits. People using plant protein, for example, lose less calcium from the bones. And because plant protein has no cholesterol and little saturated fat, a diet based on plant protein decreases the risk for heart disease.

The United States Healthy People 2010 objectives reflect the growing evidence for the health benefits of eating more plant foods. They define the key to lifelong health as eating more fruits and vegetables, whole grains, and fiber, with moderate amounts of protein and healthy fats.

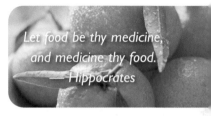

Let food be thy medicine, and medicine thy food.
—Hippocrates

But the average American consumes a diet high in processed foods and animal products and low in fruits and vegetables, whole grains, and plant proteins. Because the usual American diet typically stresses cholesterol, saturated fats, and calories, it increases our chances of heart disease, diabetes, and cancer. And the latest reports reveal that 68 percent of all American adults are either overweight or obese.[76] But with a few simple changes in what we eat, we can profoundly improve our health and lower our risk for disease.

What are the alternatives to the typical American diet? Include more fruits and vegetables in your meals by having a piece of fruit at breakfast, snacking on raw vegetables instead of crackers or chips, and making salads a part of your dinner. Have whole grains at least three times each day through eating whole wheat toast at breakfast and brown rice and beans at dinner or adding barley to your favorite vegetable soup. And don't forget nuts, seeds, and soy products. They provide excellent sources of protein without the cholesterol or saturated fats found in animal products. Such foods also have the added benefit of heart-healthy fats and compounds known as phytochemicals, which supply our bodies with the ammunition needed to protect us from most diseases. Try soy milk on your cereal, a small handful of nuts as a snack, or a soy burger the next time you barbecue. (It's really quite good!)

IT'S YOUR CHOICE

God cares about what we put into our bodies. Why? Because it's part of his great plan for us to lead healthy, productive lives as he seeks to make us whole. And recognizing this makes it just a little easier for us to begin healthy eating habits.

Water is the only drink of a wise man.
— Henry David Thoreau

Change is always difficult, especially when it comes to what we eat. We know that we should consume more fruit, but we'd much rather have a chocolate sundae for dessert. Also, we realize that eating less saturated fat and cholesterol is healthier, but when we have to work late, it's much easier to hit the drive-through for supper. Face it, convenience and taste usually win out.

Yes, altering our diet can be tough. But remember, even small adjustments can result in big health benefits. Start with something as simple as switching your afternoon snack to one-fourth cup of nuts or seeds. You'll be surprised how easy it will be to then go on to other healthy eating behaviors.

So how can you get motivated to eat healthier foods, and more important, how do you stay that way?

Sherri Flynt, a registered dietitian and co-author of the book *SuperSized Kids: How to Rescue Your Child from the Obesity Threat* offers these helpful tips for anyone wanting to make healthier food choices while maintaining a satisfying, yet balanced, diet.

- **Watch portion sizes.** Start the meal with small portions. Going back for seconds is fine, but controlling portion size can help to control calories.

- **Use small plates.** Small plates help you gain control over your portion size and trick your mind into thinking you've eaten more than you actually have.

- **Slow down!** Most adults and children not only eat too much, they eat too fast, even when they have time to relax and enjoy their food.

- **Start light.** Begin your meal with a vegetable soup, a fruit dish, or a salad.

- **Eat variety.** Variety is important because there is no single perfect food. Each food has its own unique combination of nutrients. If you vary what you eat every day, you are guaranteed a variety of nutrients.

- **Be colorful.** Pick foods with many different colors. Plant foods with lots of color —such as fruits and vegetables—are usually filled with health-giving phytochemicals. So pick natural foods that are bright red, yellow, green, orange, and blue.

- **Have breakfast.** Don't skip it. There's a reason it's called the most important meal of the day.

- **Snack healthy.** Keep a few items on hand for a fast, healthy snack during the day such as fresh fruit, ready-to-eat veggies, hummus, natural peanut butter, nuts, whole-grain crackers, raisins, or low-fat yogurt.

- **Go spare.** Serve desserts sparingly. Keep them for special occasions and see how much better you feel.

- **Find better rewards.** Resist the temptation to use food as a way to reward yourself. Food should remain a source of nourishment and enjoyment.[77]

What about animal products? Should we avoid using them entirely? When it comes to meat, poultry, and fish, Sherri recommends using them less often. "Typically we overuse meat, eating more of it than we need. We don't require that much protein, and meat usually contains the cholesterol and saturated fat associated with a higher incidence of heart disease and cancers. Minimize the amount of animal products you consume. When you minimize these foods, you want to maximize your plant foods."

For big results, Sherri also recommends starting small. "All of us are creatures of habit, and good habits take time to kick in (just as bad habits take time to overcome). Don't try to make wholesale changes in the way you eat; that's a strategy almost certain to fail. Instead, pick one or two small changes, start with them, and after you've enjoyed some success, move on and try a few more. Think 'little steps,' not 'big steps,' and you'll be far more likely to reach the destination of your dreams." [78]

A HEALTHY MOTIVATION

The apostle Paul also has a few things to say about our bodies. He talks about what God made for us as human beings. "Do you not know that your body is the temple of the Holy Spirit who is in you, whom you have from God, and you are not your own? For you were bought at a price; therefore glorify God in your body and in your spirit, which are God's" (1 Cor. 6:19–20, NKJV).

This is an extraordinary way of looking at the human body. And yet it's how God views you.

Paul doesn't say that our bodies are the shell that houses the spirit. Instead, he pictures a temple. That's something valuable. Our bodies are temples of the Holy Spirit.

Because of this, we want to take care of them. We desire to honor God by the way we treat our bodies. Why? Because God says we're that important. Obviously, our health matters to the One who made us and loves us.

As a result, we eat healthfully because we're worth it—because we're called to something noble and great. It's a motivation that can stick with us in the long run.

A NEW VIEW

Joyce began experiencing this maximum fulfillment after she made changes in her diet. "I knew that as I was getting older," she says. "I was falling into some unhealthy habits. Having a very large family and a great number of grandchildren, I love to entertain and would cook a lot as well as eat the wrong things. I knew that if I really, really believed in whole-person health, I needed to do something for myself—I had to take action.

"So I began watching the things I ate and had a more balanced diet. I began to pay more attention to what I was eating, when I was eating, and why I was eating. And it began to change me. Soon I felt better. I had energy when I woke up in the morning. When the alarm went off, I

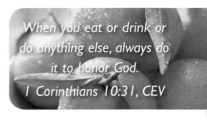

When you eat or drink or do anything else, always do it to honor God.

1 Corinthians 10:31, CEV

didn't just roll over and beg for more sleep. Many times I was awake before the alarm even sounded. I had the energy to do my very active job all day long. My weight even went down until I had lost about twenty-five pounds. At the same time my cholesterol level dropped dramatically and my skin tone improved. I just felt better about life."

EATING BETTER TO LIVE BETTER

One Christian denomination, the Adventists, have been promoting this kind of healthy eating for quite a long time now. Studies demonstrate the difference it makes. Consider, for example, the Adventist Health Study—a thirty-year investigational study on the life spans of Seventh-day Adventists living in southern California. From it we've learned that Adventists, on average, live seven to nine years longer than the general population.[79] Although we do not understand all of the reasons, it is clear that nutritional choices play a major role. Plant-based eating or using smaller amounts of animal protein lead to a longer life span and greater health during those additional years.

Looking back to the creation story, we find the original foods God gave were fruits, vegetables, whole grains, and nuts. Today, science has shown us that such foods lower our risk for heart disease, diabetes, high blood pressure, and certain cancers.

Isn't it wonderful that what God originally provided us in the Garden of Eden is just what we need today? As you plan your dietary changes, beware of gimmicks, and remember that there are no quick fixes. The key to a healthy diet, to reduction of disease, and to a longer, fuller life can be found in the garden. For more information on healthy eating be sure to check out *CREATIONHealth.com* for additional healthy eating ideas and resources.

SUCCESS STEPS

Here are three practical steps to energize your *NUTRITION* success:

MAXIMIZE—Plan foods by choosing whole grains, fruits, vegetables, legumes, and nuts. Don't constantly eat the same things. Maximize variety and color. Experiment. And maximize your taste. Enjoy your food—without this, the changes won't last.

MODERATE—Limit the amount of food you eat. Eat until you feel comfortably full and not until you are stuffed. Pay attention to your serving sizes and consider smaller, more frequent meals. Could you have five smaller meals a day instead of three larger ones? It might be worth a try. Using government recommendations as a guide (you will find them listed on most food products) is helpful. And reduce any stress when eating—eating should be a blessing and a pleasure.

MINIMIZE—Minimize animal protein intake. Minimize refined sugars and even sugar substitutes. Minimize saturated fats, which are usually solid or almost solid at room temperature. All animal fats, such as those in meat, poultry, and dairy products, are saturated. Most of the fats used in processed and fast foods are also saturated. Also, minimize the amount of salt you use. Taste your food before you shake the salt to see if it really needs any.

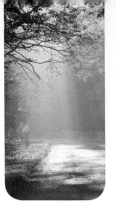

WANT TO SHARE WHAT YOU'VE LEARNED?

> **We can help you introduce the principles of CREATION Health to others in a small group setting.**

SMALL GROUPS are great for harnessing the power of CREATION Health principles in daily living. Visit the *CREATIONHealth.com* website for resources to enhance your study and discussion time. These resources are designed to strengthen behavioral changes by building relationships among participants:

- The eight-part CREATION Health Small Group Kit includes nine DVD Videos, a Small Group Leader Guide, and a Small Group Discussion Guide
- The CREATION Health Life Guides #1—8 are packed with fresh insights on abundant living linked to each of the eight CREATION Health principles

Share the Healthy Living Principles you've learned with others!

WWW.CREATIONHEALTH.COM

What does optimum health mean to you?

If you could change one unhealthy habit to a healthy one, which would it be?

When you think of "longevity," what words come to mind?

When you hear that someone died young due to poor health habits, what is your main thought?

What is your primary motivation for wanting to live a long and healthy life?

Imagine you could live to a healthy 100 years of age. What would you want to do on your 100th birthday?

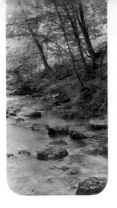

OPTIMUM HEALTH

CHAPTER 10

Loving Longevity and Living Life at Its Best

IMPROVING THE QUALITY OF OUR LIVES—THAT'S WHAT CREATION Health is all about. In the very beginning, in the book of Genesis, God gave us principles that can make all the difference. The CREATION model of health is the one with the biggest payback and the best long-term results. But we need to decide that we want this kind of life. It won't just drop into our laps or happen by accident. We must deliberately invest our time and energy into adopting such a lifestyle.

Even small decisions in many different areas will make a difference. Choosing to walk outside in the sunshine; choosing to have weekends that truly allow for rest, relaxation, and rejuvenation; choosing to think positively and to drink more water—the opportunities are endless. Your health and well-being are a journey. An old proverb states that the "journey of a thousand miles begins with the first step."

HOW TO ADD LIFE TO YOUR YEARS

Not long ago, a popular speaker named Michael was preparing to lead a seminar series in his hometown about the healing power of forgiveness.[80] The seminar was being sponsored by a local church group and was open to the public.

Although the focus of his lectures would be about relationships, he thought the people attending might enjoy hearing some tips about healthy living. So each night before the main presentation, he planned on having a special five-minute health feature. But he didn't want to do it all himself since he would be doing most of the speaking throughout the series.

> *If you want to live a long life, focus on making contributions.*
>
> *— Hans Selye*

So he searched for someone to help present the health features, and he found just the type of "unconventional" person he was looking for. Her name was Amy, and she was not a picture of perfect health. She lived off of fast food, rarely—if ever—exercised, chain-smoked, and made other questionable lifestyle choices. Though Amy attended the church on occasion with her family, it appeared she had little interest in God or spirituality. Many people in the church thought of her as a rebel, so they questioned Michael's decision to invite her to lead the nightly health features.

But Michael stood firm. He asked Amy if she would be willing to give the health segments. "I'm hoping to help people see that they can really change the direction of their health by practicing the principles of CREATION Health," he explained. "But I need an assistant, and I think you're the perfect choice."

"Me?" Amy replied. "You must be kidding. I don't live a very healthy lifestyle. Besides, I don't even know what CREATION Health is."

Michael nodded. "I know. I've been there, myself. When I was your age, nobody could tell me how to live. I was pretty unhealthy, too—though I didn't really care. It's hard to measure up to the expectations of others. But let me ask you this: If no one else were involved in this equation, would you want to live a healthy, long life, or would you want to hurt yourself by the choices you make day-by-day?"

Amy paused. "Well," she said, "I guess I would want to live long and healthy. Who wouldn't?"

"Then I was right. You are just the person to help me," Michael replied.

Several weeks before the meetings were to begin, Michael gave Amy the CREATION Health seminar material [81] and asked her to watch the DVDs and read the book, from which she was to create a five-minute health presentation for each night.

She watched the DVDs and read the CREATION Health Seminar Personal Study Guide, and sifted through the presentation slides.

As Amy prepared for her presentations, her former critics started noticing some changes. In fact, they had front-row seats to a transformation process happening right before their eyes.

She decided to stop smoking, start exercising, and to make better lifestyle choices. She even started attending church regularly, embracing the abundant life that Jesus offers, without trying to measure up to anyone else's standards.

Shortly after the series of meetings ended, Amy's employer transferred her to another state over a thousand miles away. But one of the first things she did was find a local church family she could join. She volunteered to become the leader of the church's health ministry outreach and share what she had learned about CREATION Health so others might also experience what she had experienced.

HOW TO ADD YEARS TO YOUR LIFE

Amy's story is remarkable. But what she didn't know at the time was that by adopting CREATION Health principles, she was choosing not only to add life to her years, but years to her life. How many, only God knows. But those who practice these principles have been shown to add an average of ten to fourteen years to their lifespan. [82] Even adopting a lifestyle like this in midlife can improve your health and increase your longevity. [83]

This lifestyle has been researched, documented, and verified over more than fifty years. In a special edition of *National Geographic* entitled "The Secrets of Living Longer," author Dan Buettner highlighted three major lifestyles: Okinawans in Japan, Sardinians in Italy, and Adventists in Loma Linda, California. This latter group he identified as the *All-Stars of Longevity* in America.[84] While all three groups produce longevity all-stars, the Adventist lifestyle is unique because it is the most universally transferable of the three.

This lifestyle—which you've just learned is the CREATION Health lifestyle—is worthy of practicing because:

- In many ways it's better than a pill because it has no adverse side effects.
- The results have been replicated in populations around the world.
- The results are not genetically dependent and can transfer across races and ethnic groups.
- It has produced more people who have reached one hundred years of age than any other lifestyle in America—a remarkable achievement in a culture moving in the opposite health direction today.

When many people consider a healthy living program, they tend to focus on what has to change, or what has to stop (i.e. what they have to give up). These can be strong motivators, especially in the face of debilitating illness that has been caused by wrong lifestyle choices.

However, as Amy's choices demonstrate, the strongest ongoing motivator for lifestyle change that lasts is positive—specifically, the desire to live life to the full, in order to serve God and humanity better. For when we align our lifestyle choices with a powerful purpose or sense of calling on our lives, we are able to tap into the positive power of hope.

How many years could you add to your life by practicing the principles of CREATION Health? Why not set a goal of living a healthy and productive one hundred years of age? That's what one of my other books is about. It's called *8 Secrets of a Healthy 100*, and its vision keeps me inspired day by day. Sometimes I imagine living long enough and healthy enough to bring this message, which is really God's message, to the world and to the fourth and fifth generations of my family. I invite you to ponder the impact you could have on your family and the world as a result of living to a healthy 100, yourself. Just imagine!

ADD OTHERS TO YOUR COMPANY OF COMRADES

If I had a cure for heart disease, cancer, high blood pressure—okay for *any chronic disease*—and I refused to share it with humankind, what would you think of me? You'd probably argue that I had a *moral obligation* to spread that news worldwide.

Well, the principles of CREATION Health are the closest we can come to those kind of "cures," and my moral obligation to share what I know is actually what drives me to tell you—and anyone who will listen—about CREATION Health.

And people will listen, because these days just about everyone, from your neighbor to your pastor to your boss to your doctor to your governor, is aware that Ben Franklin's axiom applies now more than ever: "An ounce of prevention is worth a pound of cure."

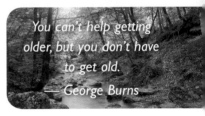

You can't help getting older, but you don't have to get old.
— George Burns

In fact, businesses are joining our effort to promote healthy living through the CREATION Health program. Why? Well, some are motivated altruistically; in other words, they want to give their employees their best possible chance at living well and long. But their bottom line benefits also: healthier workers equals happier workers, lower healthcare costs, and greater productivity.

State and local governments are also endorsing and using the principles of CREATION Health. They're bringing the CREATION Health seminar to their employees, using it in their communities, and sending people to our website: CREATIONHealth.com so they can learn more about how to live life to the fullest.

We've also developed a CREATION Health curriculum and other materials for use in schools. Now students in elementary school, high school, and college will have the opportunity to learn the principles of whole-person health that can last a lifetime.

And we've launched a movement among churches. Our goal is to equip health-conscious churches to establish a health ministry designed not only to educate their members, but to offer information to their neighbors and communities that is timely and relevant, scientifically based, biblically sound, yet still nonthreatening. It's a powerful idea that goes beyond denominational boundaries because healthier living is really God's idea and his original design all the way back to the Garden of Eden.

> If we don't change, we don't grow. If we don't grow, we aren't really living.
> — Gail Sheehy

While I'd like to share many interesting stories of how CREATION Health is being used creatively in businesses, hospitals, local governments, schools, and churches, let me conclude by sharing Barbara's experience with you. Barbara is a Health Ministry team leader at her church, and she shared these stories of how lives have been changed by this unique focus on health.

She wrote, "After completing the CREATION Health session on Environment, one of our staff pastors redecorated his office area. New paint was applied, calming pictures of nature were hung, and decorations reflected a positive, balanced environment. During the following weeks, not only did the pastor enjoy his new surroundings, but all of the guests who met with him felt the positive influence of a great environment. His office is a welcoming and peaceful place to meet and a great example of how changing your environment influences everyday life!"

Barbara added, "Then one of our staff members decided to revamp their eating habits after the CREATION Health session on Nutrition.

She has lost twenty-five pounds and feels great! This change in lifestyle has resulted in her whole family eating healthier and everyone feeling better emotionally as well as physically."

Today, you can be at the forefront of helping your church, business, school, or community experience the benefits of wholistic health. The principles of CREATION Health are not new. They are as old as humanity, going back to the story of creation. But they can seem new to anyone raised in a culture that thrives on "fast everything," from fast food to fast lifestyle to fast satisfaction of our every whim.

The "discovery" that is part of CREATION Health is that these God-given principles for living life to the full really do satisfy today's needs. While no one can guarantee who will live to see one hundred, it's the spirit that matters. As Abraham Lincoln said, "It's not the years in your life that count. It's the life in your years."

Your outlook and choices are key, but the other principles are also integral to achieving and maintaining optimal health. Every positive choice makes the next one easier. As good results multiply, you gain momentum. You start feeling better and looking better. And there will come a time when you won't return to that old lifestyle for anything.

The CREATION Health model is showing the way. Make that journey, starting right now, with God at your side. Put into practice the principles you've learned—principles established by God and supported by medical science. You'll be giving a gift to yourself in body, mind, and spirit. You'll also be offering a marvelous gift to your loved ones—the gift of a happier, healthier them.

About the Authors

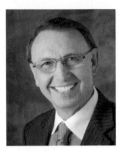

DES CUMMINGS JR., PHD, serves as president of the Florida Hospital Foundation and executive vice president for Florida Hospital, the largest admitting hospital in America. Dr. Cummings holds a PhD degree in leadership and management with emphasis in statistical forecasting. Dr. Cummings also holds a master of divinity degree and is an ordained minister.

Motivated by a vision to help people live to a Healthy 100, Dr. Cummings gave leadership to the development of Celebration Health, a showcase hospital in the Disney city of Celebration, Florida. This facility has attracted national and international attention as a model of health and healing for the twenty-first century.

Dr. Cummings is committed to the concept of empowering patients to take charge of their health and distributing medical knowledge into the community. Dr. Cummings is the author or coauthor of four books, including *CREATION Health Discovery* (over 750,000 in print). He speaks to national and international conferences on the future of healthcare, specializing in strategies for whole-person care, healthy communities, and the hospital of the future. It is his belief that we must recreate a new vision of American healthcare for the twenty-first century that is financially viable and enhances quality of life for all Americans. This task calls for the very best thinking of the brightest minds in American healthcare.

In the Cummings home, health and healing is a family affair. Dr. Cummings' wife, Mary Lou, is a nurse and health educator who gave leadership to the development of the Florida Hospital Parish Nurse program and Women's Center at Celebration Health. She has also been an active contributor to the Healthy 100 vision. The Cummings live in Celebration, Florida. They have two adult children, Tracy and Derek, a wonderful son-in-law and daughter-in-law, Denis and Nalani, and two amazing grandchildren, Kelsey and DJ. For more information, visit *DesCummings.com*.

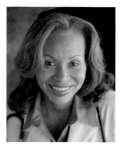

MONICA REED, MD, serves as Chief Executive Officer (CEO) of Florida Hospital Celebration Health—a facility recognized by the Wall Street Journal as the "Hospital of the Future." As a physician, speaker, author, medical news reporter, and hospital administrator, Dr. Reed has dedicated her professional career to promoting health, healing, and wellness. Dr. Reed has filled many other key roles at Florida Hospital in her career, including: senior medical officer—overseeing the relationship between the hospital and its two thousand physicians; medical director for the Celebration Health Center for Women's Medicine; and associate director of the Family Practice Residency Program.

Dr. Reed is the author or coauthor of seven books. She has served as a medical news reporter in Orlando, Florida, and Huntsville, Alabama. In 2008, Dr. Reed was named one of Modern Healthcare's Top 25 Minority Executives in Healthcare.

Dr. Reed is married to Stanton Reed. They have two daughters, Melanie and Megan. For more information, visit *CREATIONHealthBreakthrough.com.*

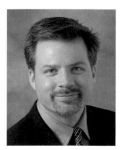

TODD CHOBOTAR serves as founder, publisher, and editor-in-chief of the Florida Hospital publishing program. The focus of his work is creating consumer books, professional monographs, and other resources. He is the author or coauthor of four books and has served as editor on dozens of publications. Chobotar holds two business degrees from Andrews University. He lives in Orlando with his wife, Jeannine, twins Joshua and Sarah, and two cats Simon & Schuster. For more information, visit *ToddChobotar.com.*

About the Publisher

The CREATION Health model is the foundation of the Adventist Health System. These eight principles have been practiced by hundreds of thousands of people over the last century and have resulted in national studies concluding that following these principles can add ten to fourteen years to your life. These studies have also demonstrated that following the eight principles brings about a significant reduction in the risk of lifestyle diseases such as cancer, stroke, and heart disease. By following the CREATION Health principles, Adventists have become known as the healthiest people in the world.

The story behind this remarkable journey began in 1863 when James White, then president of the young Seventh-day Adventist Church, suffered a series of mini-strokes that made it impossible for him to serve in his leadership role. Rather than accept the normal treatments of the day, James and his wife, Ellen, chose to search Scripture for a biblical model of health. They found it in the Genesis story of creation. As they examined God's original design for Adam and Eve in the Garden of Eden, James and Ellen discovered God's principles of whole-person health.

After eighteen months of carefully following the CREATION Health model, James White was back to good health and, along with his wife, was sharing these principles at every opportunity. In 1866 several key members of the church's executive committee were so ill that they could not meet. The members who could attend the meeting chose to make health the number-one item on their agenda. That day the church leaders made a commitment to build "sanitariums" that would combine the best of science with the best of faith, and treat patients with the compassion that Christ showed during his healing ministry. This combination of science and faith wrapped in compassion is the foundation for the healing ministry of the Adventist Health System.

Six months later, the church opened the Western Health Reform Institute (later renamed Battle Creek Sanitarium) in Battle Creek, Michigan. It proved to be a remarkably successful enterprise. At the height of its popularity, the Battle Creek Sanitarium was the health destination for America. It accommodated 1,500 patients and attracted the best-known people of the day. Henry Ford, Thomas Edison, J.C. Penney, Clara Barton, George Bernard Shaw, John D. Rockefeller Jr., Dale Carnegie, and Amelia Earhart are all listed on the patient rosters. They, and hundreds of others, came to Battle Creek to recuperate from the stress and intemperance of their busy lives.

One of the sanitarium's biggest attractions was its charismatic medical director, Dr. John Harvey Kellogg. Dr. Kellogg was a skillful physician, an advocate of a healthy vegetarian diet, and a proponent of God's principles of whole-person health. It was at Battle Creek that Kellogg and his brother, W.K. Kellogg, developed breakfast cereals, including granola and corn flakes, as alternatives to the high-fat biscuit-and-gravy, bacon-and-egg breakfasts that most Americans were eating. Dr. Kellogg traveled the world speaking on the benefits of healthful living, and searching for better approaches to healing. Dr. Kellogg studied surgery under some of the world's leading physicians, and as anesthesia was perfected for use in surgery, he brought this new science to Battle Creek.

The success of the healthcare at Battle Creek led the Seventh-day Adventist leaders to develop additional medical facilities. In the next twenty years the church opened forty facilities, including hospitals and medical schools, around the world. The success of those facilities, and the health focus of thousands of physicians, dentists, nurses, and other caregivers can easily be attributed to Dr. Kellogg's fundamental commitment to the CREATION Health model of health and healing.

Today, with more than 500 hospitals, clinics, and healthcare centers around the world, the healthcare ministry of the Seventh-day Adventist church continues to infuse the CREATION Health concepts with the best of science and medical technology. For us, Jesus Christ is the master physician who guides all that we do. In the tradition of Dr. Kellogg, we believe that whole-person healing requires a combination of science and faith wrapped in compassion.

Adventist Health System is one portion of the Seventh-day Adventist healthcare system around the world. To learn more about our hospitals, rehab centers, assisted living centers, nursing homes, and community health programs, all operated within the life-transforming message of CREATION Health, please visit the website *AdventistHealthSystem.com.*

Acknowledgements

THIS BOOK IS BASED ON THE PREMISE THAT THE model for health is embedded in the creation story found in the Bible. By applying these eight principles that God built into the Garden of Eden we can experience "optimum vitality." My wife, Mary Lou, has helped me to actualize these principles in my life and demonstrated how they can be designed into a care model for the Women's Center at Celebration Health.

My deep appreciation is due to Monica Reed, MD, who implemented these principles as the first medical director of the Women's Center at Celebration Health and continues to promote them now as CEO of Celebration Health. Her insights on this book have been invaluable.

My work at Florida Hospital has been among the most rewarding experiences of my life. I would like to thank Tom Werner and Don Jernigan, PhD, for their unwavering support and encouragement. Without their visionary leadership, Celebration Health and the CREATION Health model wouldn't be what they are today. Lars Houmann and Brian Paradis have had a lasting impact on my life and helped me to shape many of the ideas in this book. We worked together for more than three years to implement these principles at Celebration Health.

I owe a special debt of thanks to the team who helped create the vision of the CREATION Health principles. My sincere thanks are due to Ted Hamilton, MD, who wrote the original philosophy statement; Dr. Dick Tibbits, who coached the health professionals in implementing it; and Kevin Edgerton, who developed the communications materials to popularize it. I would like to thank contributors Steve Mosley, Dick Duerksen, Dr. George Guthrie, Sherri Flynt, Susan Sipprell, Simon Lia, Stacy Nelson, and Lorraine Zima-Lenon.

Special thanks to the publishing team who worked so hard to bring this book to life: Todd Chobotar, Dr. David Biebel, Lillian Boyd, Stephanie Lind, and Laurel Prizigley.

End Notes

1 Mette Andresen, Ulla Runge, et al. "Perceived Autonomy and Activity Choices Among Physically Disabled Older People in Nursing Home Settings: A Randomized Trial," *Journal of Aging and Health* 21, no. 8 (2009), 1133–1158.

2 Judith Rodin and Ellen J. Langer, "Long-Term Effects of a Control-Relevant Intervention with the Institutionalized Aged," *Journal of Personality and Social Psychology* 35, no. 12 (1977), 897–902. http://capital2.capital.edu/faculty/jfournie/documents/Rodin_Judith.pdf.

3 J.M. Koolhaas, S.M. Korte, S.F. De Boer, B.J. Van Der Vegt et al., "Coping Styles in Animals: Current Status in Behavior and Stress-Physiology," *Neuroscience and Biobehavioral Reviews* 23, no. 7 (November 1999), 925–35. http://dx.doi.org/10.1016/S0149-7634(99)00026-3.

4 This arena of study has greatly expanded since the Koolhaas article was published. An extensive analysis was published in *The Ethics of Research Involving Animals*, published by the Nuffield Council on Bioethics (London, 2005). Of particular relevance is chapter 4 of this document, available online free, in PDF format at: http://www.nuffieldbioethics.org/sites/default/files/The%20ethics%20of%20research%20involving%20animals%20-%20full%20report.pdf.

5 Jennifer A. Mains and Forrest R. Scogin, "The Effectiveness of Self-administered Treatments: A Practice-friendly Review of the Research," *Journal of Clinical Psychology* 59, no. 2 (Feb. 2003), 237–46. DOI: 10.1002/jclp.10145. Also see: "The Development and Safe Use of Patient-Controlled Analgesia" (Editorial) *The British Journal of Anesthesiology* 68, no. 4, 331–332.

6 Viktor E. Frankl, *Man's Search for Meaning* (Boston, MA: Beacon Press, 2006), 66.

7 As quoted in David Katz and Maura González, *Way to Eat: A Six-Step Path to Lifelong Weight Control* (Naperville, IL: Sourcebooks, 2002), 34. See also: http://www.hhs.gov/ohrp/archive/irb/irb_chapter3.htm.

8 Celia B. Fisher and Richard M. Lerner, eds., *Encyclopedia of Applied Developmental Science, Volume 1*, (Thousand Oaks, CA: Sage Publications, Inc., 2005), 325.

9 Katz and González, *Way to Eat*, 35.

10 Penelope A. Bryant, John Trinder, and Nigel Curtis, "Sick and Tired: Does Sleep Have a Vital Role in the Immune System?" *Nature Reviews Immunology* 4 (June 2004): 457–467. DOI:10.1038/nri1369.

11 Tiffany Field, "Infant Massage," Chap. 7 in *Touch* (Cambridge, MA: The MIT Press, 2001).

12 James B. Maas, *Power Sleep* (New York: Harper Collins, 1998), 14.

13 Visit: www.heartmath.com, and see the book by Doc Childre and Deborah Rozman, *Transforming Anxiety: The HeartMath Solution for Overcoming Fear and Worry and Creating Serenity* (Oakland, CA: New Harbinger Publications, 2006), 104–05.

14 John Newman, *How to Stay Cool, Calm & Collected When the Pressure's On* (New York: AMACON, 1992), 85.

15 Scott Brady, *Pain Free for Life: The 6-Week Cure for Chronic Pain—Without Surgery or Drugs* (New York: Center Street, 2006).

16 Guy H. Montgomery, Dana H. Bovbjerg, "The Development of Anticipatory Nausea in Patients Receiving Adjuvant Chemotherapy for Breast Cancer" *Physiology & Behavior*, 61, no. 5 (May 1997), 737–741. See: http://www.sciencedirect.com/science/article/pii/S0031938496005288.

17 Aileen Ludington and Hans Diehl, *Health Power: Health by Choice Not Chance* (Newport, WA: White Horse Media, 2011), 194–97.

18   Takashi Oyabu, Ayako Sawada, Takishi Onodera, Kozaburo Takaneka, and Bill Wolverton, "Characteristics of Potted Plants for Removing Offensive Odors," *Sensor and Actuators B: Chemical* 89, no. 1 and 2 (March 2003): 131–36. http://dx.doi.org/10.1016/S0925-4005(02)00454-9.

19   "Inspirational Quotes," Steven Halpern, accessed January 28, 2012, http://www.inspirationalquotes4u.com/stress/index.html.

20   "Quotations Book," Luigi Russolo, accessed January 28, 2012, http://quotationsbook.com/quote/28251/.

21   "The Quotations Page," Elizabeth Sitwell, accessed January 28, 2012, http://www.quotationspage.com / quote/1526.html.

22   Field, *Touch*, 10.

23   Kathleen C. Light, Karen M. Grewen, and Janet A. Amico, "More Frequent Partner Hugs and Higher Oxytocin Levels are Linked to Lower Blood Pressure and Heart Rate in Premenopausal Women," *Biological Psychology* 69, no. 1 (April 2005): 5–21. http://dx.doi.org/10.1016/j.biopsycho.2004.11.002.

24   James L Halliday, *Psychosocial Medicine: A Study of the Sick Society* (New York: Norton, 1948).

25   "Brainy Quote," Virginia Satir, accessed January 28, 2012, http://www.brainyquote.com/quotes / quotes/v/virginiasa175185.html.

26   Source: "Physical Activity for Everyone: The Benefits of Physical Activity" (Feb. 16, 2011). Posted online at: http://www.cdc.gov/physicalactivity/everyone/health/index.html.

27   See: http://www.lifeshealthcare.com/2011/12/regular-exercise-makes-sleep-more.html. For the positive effect of exercise on sleep in patients receiving radiation, see: Lisa K. Sprod, Oxana G. Palesh, Michelle C. Janelsins, Luke J. Peppone, Charles E. Heckler et al., "Exercise, Sleep Quality, and Mediators of Sleep in Breast and Prostate Cancer Patients Receiving Radiation Therapy," *Community Oncology* 7, no. 10 (October 2010): 463–71, http://www.ncbi.nlm.nih.gov/pmc/articles/PMC3026283/.

28   C.B. Taylor, J.F. Sallis, and R. Needle, "The Relation of Physical Activity and Exercise to Mental Health," *Public Health Reports* 100, no. 2 (Mar–Apr 1985): 195–202, http://www.ncbi.nlm.nih.gov/pmc/articles / PMC1424736/.

29   "Fewer Americans Smoke, but Fewer Physically Active in Leisure-Time," Centers for Disease Control and Prevention, updated June 29, 2005, http://www.cdc.gov/nchs/pressroom/05facts/earlyre-lease200506.htm.

30   "Fitness at Any Age," Medicinenet.com, accessed January 29, 2012, http://www.medicinenet.com/exercise_and_activity/article.htm.

31   Queen's University, "Physical Fitness Cuts Men's Heart Disease Risk In Half, New Queen's Study Shows," ScienceDaily (September 4, 2005), retrieved January 29, 2012, http://www.sciencedaily.com / releases/2005/09/050904122600.htm.

32   Steven N. Blair, James B. Kampert, Harold W. Kohl III, Carolyn E. Barlow, Caroline A. Macera et al., "Influences of Cardiorespiratory Fitness and Other Precursors on Cardiovascular Disease and All-Cause Mortality in Men and Women," *JAMA* 276, no. 3 (1996): 205–10, DOI: 10.1001/jama.1996.03540030039029.

33   Taylor, Sallis, and Needle, "The Relation of Physical Activity and Exercise to Mental Health," *Public Health Reports*, 195–202.

34   Dennis Patrick O'Hara, "Is There a Role for Prayer and Spirituality in Health Care?" *Medical Clinics of North America* 86, no. 1 (January 2002): 33–46, http://dx.doi.org/10.1016/S0025-7125(03)00070-1.

35   Jason Schnittker, "When is Faith Enough? The Effects of Religious Involvement on Depression," *Journal for the Scientific Study of Religion* 40, no. 3 (September 2001): 393–411. DOI: 10.1111/0021-8294.00065.

36   Kate Miriam Loewenthal, Marco Cinnirella, Georgina Evdoka, and Paula Murphy, "Faith Conquers All? Beliefs About the Role of Religious Factors in Coping with Depression Among Different Cultural-religious Groups in the UK," *British Journal of Medical Psychology* 74, no. 3 (September 2001): 293–303. DOI: 10.1348/000711201160993.

37   David B. Biebel and Harold G. Koenig, *New Light on Depression* (Grand Rapids, MI: Zondervan, 2004), 263, 270.

38   Lloyd Pickering, "Hellfire, Home, and Harm: An Investigation of the Interaction Between Religiosity, Family Processes, and Adolescent Deviant Behavior," Auburn University Theses and Dissertations, May 15, 2005, http://hdl.handle.net/10415/1005.

39   Source: Drs. Alex Bunn and David Randall, "Health Benefits of Christian Faith" (Christian Medical Fellowship; London, England, 2011), CMF Files no: 44.

40   Dale Matthews, *The Faith Factor: Proof of the Healing Power of Prayer* (New York: Penguin, 1998), 16.

41   Adapted from *If God Is So Good, Why Do I Hurt So Bad?* (Orlando, FL: Florida Hospital Publishing, 2014).

42   Sheldon Cohen, Lynn G. Underwood, and Benjamin H. Gottlieb, *Social Support Measurement and Intervention: A Guide for Health and Social Scientists* (New York: Oxford Press, 2000).

43   David Spiegel, Helena C. Kraemer, Joan R. Bloom, and Ellen Gottheil, "Effect of Psychosocial Treatment on Survival of Patients with Metastatic Breast Cancer," *Lancet* 334, no. 8668 (October 1989): 888–891, http://dx.doi.org/10.1016/S0140-6736(89)91551-1.

44   F.I. Fawzy, N.W. Fawzy, C.S. Hyun, R. Elashoff, D. Guthrie et al., "Malignant Melanoma. Effects of an Early Structured Psychiatric Intervention, Coping, and Affective State on Recurrence and Survival 6 Years Later," *Archives of General Psychiatry* 50, no. 9 (September 1993): 681–89, http://www.ncbi.nlm.nih.gov/pubmed/8357293.

45   James S. House, "Social Isolation Kills, But How and Why?" *Psychosomatic Medicine* 63, no. 2 (March 2001): 273–274, http://www.psychosomaticmedicine.org/content/63/2/273.short.

46   "The Roseto Effect," accessed January 31, 2012, http://www.uic.edu/classes/osci/osci590 /14_2%20 The%20Roseto%20Effect.htm.

47   Dean Ornish, *Love and Survival: 8 Pathways to Intimacy and Health* (New York: HarperCollins, 1998), 2–3, 14.

48   Dara Sorkin, Karen S. Rook, and John L. Lu, "Loneliness, Lack of Emotional Support, Lack of Companionship, and the Likelihood of Having a Heart Condition in an Elderly Sample," *Annals of Behavioral Medicine* 24, no. 4 (2002): 290–98, DOI: 10.1207/S15324796ABM2404_05.

49   Buck Wolf, "The Miracle Hug Lady," ABC News.com, July 12, 2011, http://abcnews.go.com / Entertainment/WolfFiles/story?id=92869&page=1.

50   Herdley Paolini, PhD, *Inside the Mind of a Physician: Illuminating the Mystery of How Doctors Think, What They Feel, and Why They Do the Things They Do* (Orlando: Florida Hospital Publishing, 2009).

51   Melissa A. Rosenkranz, Daren C. Jackson, Kim M. Dalton, Isa Dolski, Carol D. Ryff et al., "Affective Style and In Vivo Immune Response: Neurobehavioral Mechanisms," *Proceedings of the National Academy of Sciences* 100 (2003):11148–52, http://psyphz.psych.wisc.edu/web/pubs/2003/Style_immune_response.pdf.

52   Julienne E. Bower, Margaret E. Kemeny, Shelley E. Taylor, and John L. Fahey, "Cognitive Processing, Discovery of Meaning, CD4 Decline, and AIDS-related Mortality Among Bereaved HIV-seropositive Men," *Journal of Consulting and Clinical Psychology* 66, no.6 (Dec 1998): 979–86, DOI: 10.1037/0022-006X.66.6.979.

53   Michael D. Lemonick, "How Your Mind Can Heal Your Body," *Special Issue Time Magazine*, January 20, 2003, http://www.hypnosis.edu/articles/power-of-mind.

54   Dominique L. Musselman, Dwight L. Evans, Charles B. Nemeroff, "The Relationship of Depression to Cardiovascular Disease: Epidemiology, Biology, and Treatment," *Archives of General Psychiatry* 55, no. 7 (July 1998): 580–92, http://archpsyc.ama-assn.org/cgi/content/abstract/55/7/580.

55   B.J.J. Abdullah, "Learning How to Learn," *Biomedical Imaging and Intervention Journal* 4, no. 1 (2008): e10, DOI: 10.2349/biij.4.1.e10.

56   Patrick J. Lustman and Ray E. Clouse, "Depression in Diabetic Patients: The Relationship Between Mood and Glycemic Control," *Journal of Diabetes and Its Complications* 19, no. 2 (March 2005): 113–22, http://www.jdcjournal.com/article/S1056-8727(04)00004-2/abstract.

57   Giovanni Cizza, Svetlana Primma, and Gyorgy Csako, "Depression as a Risk Factor for Osteoporosis," *Trends in Endocrinology and Metabolism* 20, no. 8 (October 2009): 367–73, http://dx.doi.org/10.1016/j.tem.2009.05.003.

58   Lemonick, "How Your Mind Can Heal Your Body," *Time*.

59   Redford Williams and Virginia Williams, *Anger Kills: 17 Strategies for Controlling the Hostility That Can Harm Your Health* (New York: HarperCollins, 1993). For an updated analysis, see: Timothy W. Smith, Kelly Grazer, et al, "Hostility, Anger, Aggressiveness, and Coronary Heart Disease: An Interpersonal Perspective on Personality, Emotion, and Health," *Journal of Personality*, 72, no. 6 (2004), 1217–1270.

60   Geoffrey Cowley, "Our Bodies, Our Fears," *Newsweek*, February 24, 2003, http://www.articlesfactory.com /articles/science/our-bodies-our-fears.html.

61   Geoffrey Cowley, "Newsweek Cover: Anxiety and Your Brain," *Newsweek*, February 24, 2003, http://www.prnewswire.com/news-releases/newsweek-cover-anxiety-and-your-brain-74367212.html.

62   Cowley, "Our Bodies, Our Fears," *Newsweek*.

63   Martin Seligman, *Helplessness: On Depression, Development, and Death* (San Francisco: W.H. Freeman, 1975). For later information related to this theme, see: Laura D. Kubzansky, PhD, David Sparrow, DSc, Pantel Vokonas, MD, and Ichiro Kawachi, MD, "Is the Glass Half Empty or Half Full? A Prospective Study of Optimism and Coronary Heart Disease in the Normative Aging Study," *Psychosomatic Medicine 63, no. 6* (2001), 910–916. Summary: An optimistic explanatory style may protect against risk of coronary heart disease in older men. Posted at: http://www.psychosomaticmedicine.org/content/63/6/910.short.

64   Frankl, *Man's Search for Meaning*.

65   Adapted from *52 Ways to Feel Great Today*, by Drs. David B. Biebel and James E. Dill, and Bobbie Dill, RN (Orlando, FL: Florida Hospital Publishing, 2012), 136–139.

66   Loren L. Toussaint, David R. Williams, Marc A. Musick, and Susan A. Everson, "Forgiveness and Health: Age Differences in a U.S. Probability Sample," *Journal of Adult Development* 8, no. 4 (2001): 249–57, DOI: 10.1023/A:1011394629736.

67   Michael J. McFarland, Cheryl A. Smith, Loren L. Toussaint, and Patricia A. Thomas, "Forgiveness of Others and Health: Do Race and Neighborhood Matter?" *Journals of Gerontology: Series B* 67B, no. 1 (2012): 66–75. DOI: 10.1093/geronb/gbr121.

68   Dick Tibbits and Steve Halliday, *Forgive to Live: How Forgiveness Can Save Your Life* (Orlando, FL: Florida Hospital Publishing, 2006).

69   Ron Hoggan and James Braly, "Food Allergies and Depression: How Modern Eating Habits May Contribute to Depression," About.com, updated August 26, 2011, http://depression.about.com/cs/diet/a/foodallergies.htm.

70   See article: http://articles.baltimoresun.com/1992-06-15/news/1992167007_1_diets-regeneration-cell.

71   David C. Nieman, Dru A. Henson, Lucille L. Smith, Alan C. Utter, Debra M. Vinci et al., "Cytokine Changes After a Marathon Race," *Journal of Applied Physiology* 91, no. 1 (July 2001): 109–14, http://jap. physiology.org /content/91/1/109.short.

72 · Many studies are being conducted on this subject: For one report, see *Medicine & Science in Sports & Exercise, 41, no. 1* (Jan. 2009), 155–163. View summary at: http://journals.lww.com/acsm-msse/pages/ articleviewer.aspx?year=2009&issue=01000&article=00018&type=abstract.

73   M.L. Slattery, D.R. Jacobs Jr, J.E. Hilner, B.J. Caan, L. Van Horn et al., "Meat Consumption and its Associations with Other Diet and Health Factors in Young Adults: The CARDIA Study," *American Journal of Clinical Nutrition* 54, no. 5 (November 1991): 930–35, http://www.ajcn.org/content/54/5/930. short.

74   See: Winston J Craig, "Health Effects of Vegan Diets," *American Journal of Clinical Nutrition* 89, no. 5 (May 2009): 1627S–33S, DOI: 10.3945/ajcn.2009.26736N.

75   S. Rajaram and J. Sabaté, "Fifth International Congress on Vegetarian Nutrition," *American Journal of Clinical Nutrition* 89, no. 5 (May 2009): 1541S–42S, http://www.ncbi.nlm.nih.gov/pubmed/19279078.

76   "Obesity and Overweight," Centers for Disease Control and Prevention, updated November 17, 2011, http://www.cdc.gov/nchs/fastats/overwt.htm.

77   Adapted from: Walt Larimore, Sherri Flynt, Steve Halliday, *SuperSized Kids: How to Rescue Your Child From the Obesity Threat* (New York: Center Street, 2005), 178, 182–183.

78   Ibid.,

79   "The Adventist Health Study: Related Investigations and Future Plans," Loma Linda University School of Public Health, accessed February 2, 2012, http://www.llu.edu/public-health/health/future.page.

80   The name of the seminar was "Forgive to Live" by Dr. Dick Tibbits. For more information about this program, visit www.ForgiveToLive.net.

81   If you would like more information about the CREATION Health seminar material—including the CREATION Health Seminar Personal Study Guide and DVD series—turn to the Resources section at the end of this book or visit www.CREATIONHealth.com.

82   Tom LeDuc, "The Adventist Contribution to Global Health," part of a larger article entitled "The Adventists and What They Mean to You." on www.WorldLifeExpectancy.com. See: http://www.world-lifeexpectancy.com/what-adventists-mean-to-you. Accessed July 15, 2011.

83   Dana E. King, MD, et al. "Turning Back the Clock: Adopting a Healthy Lifestyle in Middle Age." *The American Journal of Medicine* (2007) 120, 598–603.

84   Dan Buettner, "The Secrets of Long Life," *National Geographic* (November 2005): 2–26.

LEAD YOUR COMMUNITY
TO HEALTHY
LIVING

CREATIONHealth.com

Shop online for CREATION Health Seminars, Books, & Resources

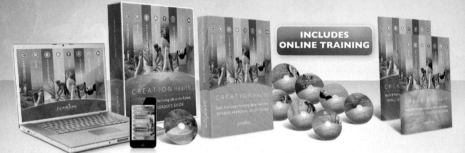

INCLUDES ONLINE TRAINING

Seminar Leader Kit
Everything a leader needs to conduct this seminar successfully, including key questions to facilitate group discussion and PowerPoint™ presentations for each of the eight principles.

Participant Guide
A study guide with essential information from each of the eight lessons along with outlines, self-assessments, and questions for people to fill in as they follow along.

Small Group Kit
It's easy to lead a small group using the CREATION Health videos, the Small Group Leader Guide, and the Small Group Discussion Guide.

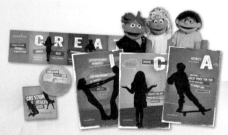

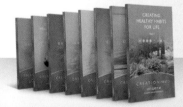

CREATION Kids
CREATION Health Kids can make a big difference in homes, schools, and congregations. Lead kids in your community to healthier, happier living.

Life Guide Series
These guides include questions designed to help individuals or small groups study the depths of every principle and learn strategies for integrating them into everyday life.

GUIDES AND ASSESSMENTS

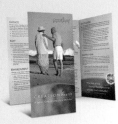

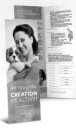

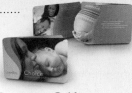

Pregnancy Guides
Expert advice on how to be CREATION Healthy while expecting.

Senior Guide
Share the CREATION Health principles with seniors and help them be healthier and happier as they live life to the fullest.

Self-Assessment
This instrument raises awareness about how CREATION Healthy a person is in each of the eight major areas of wellness.

Pocket Guide
A tool for keeping people committed to living all of the CREATION Health principles daily.

Tote Bag
A convenient way for bringing CREATION Health materials to and from class.

Tumbler
Practice good Nutrition and keep yourself hydrated with a CREATION Health tumbler in an assortment of fun colors.

MARKETING MATERIALS

Postcards, Posters, Stationery, and more
You can effectively advertise and generate community excitement about your CREATION Health seminar with a wide range of available marketing materials such as enticing postcards, flyers, posters, and more.

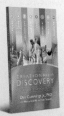

Bible Stories
God is interested in our physical, mental, and spiritual well-being. Throughout the Bible you can discover the eight principles for full life.

CREATION HEALTH BOOKS

CREATION Health Discovery
Written by Des Cummings Jr., PhD, Monica Reed, MD, and Todd Chobotar, this wonderful companion resource introduces people to the CREATION Health philosophy and lifestyle.

CREATION Health Devotional
In this devotional you will discover stories about experiencing God's grace in the tough times, God's delight in triumphant times, and God's presence in peaceful times.

English: Hardcover
Spanish: Softcover

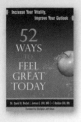

52 Ways to Feel Great Today (Softcover)

Wouldn't you love to feel great today? Changing your outlook and injecting energy into your day often begins with small steps. In *52 Ways to Feel Great Today*, you'll discover an abundance of simple, inexpensive, fun things you can do to make a big difference in how you feel today and every day. Tight on time? No problem. Each chapter is written as a short, easy-to-implement idea.

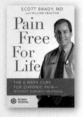

Pain Free For Life (Hardcover)

In *Pain Free For Life*, Scott C. Brady, MD,—founder of Florida Hospital's Brady Institute for Health—shares for the first time with the general public his dramatically successful solution for chronic back pain, fibromyalgia, chronic headaches, irritable bowel syndrome, and other "impossible to cure" pains. Dr. Brady leads pain-racked readers to a pain-free life using powerful mind-body-spirit strategies used at the Brady Institute—where more than 80 percent of his chronic-pain patients have achieved 80–100 percent pain relief within weeks.

If Today Is All I Have (Softcover)

At its heart, Linda's captivating account chronicles the struggle to reconcile her three dreams of experiencing life as a "normal woman" with the tough realities of her medical condition. Her journey is punctuated with insights that are at times humorous, painful, provocative, and life-affirming.

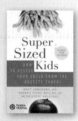

SuperSized Kids (Hardcover)

In *SuperSized Kids*, Walt Larimore, MD, and Sherri Flynt, MPH, RD, LD, show how the mushrooming childhood obesity epidemic is destroying children's lives, draining family resources, and pushing America dangerously close to a total healthcare collapse—while also explaining, step by step, how parents can work to avert the coming crisis by taking control of the weight challenges facing every member of their family.

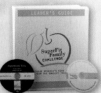

SuperFit Family Challenge – Leader's Guide

Perfect for your community, church, small group, or other settings.
The SuperFit Family Challenge Leader's Guide Includes:
- Eight weeks of pre-designed PowerPoint™ presentations.
- Professionally designed marketing materials and group handouts from direct mailers to reading guides.
- Training directly from Author Sherri Flynt, MPH, RD, LD, across six audio CDs.
- Media coverage and FAQ on DVD.

Forgive To Live (English: Hardcover / Spanish: Softcover)

In *Forgive to Live* Dr. Tibbits presents the scientifically proven steps for forgiveness—taken from the first clinical study of its kind conducted by Stanford University and Florida Hospital.

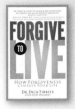

Forgive To Live Workbook (Softcover)

This interactive guide will show you how to forgive – insight by insight, step by step—in a workable plan that can effectively reduce your anger, improve your health, and put you in charge of your life again, no matter how deep your hurts.

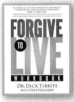

Forgive To Live Devotional (Hardcover)

In his powerful new devotional, Dr. Dick Tibbits reveals the secret to forgiveness. This compassionate devotional is a stirring look at the true meaning of forgiveness. Each of the fifty-six spiritual insights includes motivational Scripture, an inspirational prayer, and two thought-provoking questions. The insights are designed to encourage your journey as you begin to *Forgive to Live*.

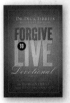

Forgive To Live God's Way, A Small Group Resource (Softcover)

Forgiveness is so important that our very lives depend on it. Churches teach us that we should forgive, but how do you actually learn to forgive? In this spiritual workbook, noted author, psychologist, and ordained minister Dr. Dick Tibbits takes you step-by-step through an eight-week forgiveness format that is easy to understand and follow.

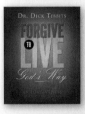

Forgive To Live Leader's Guide

Perfect for your community, church, small group, or other settings.
The Forgive To Live Leader's Guide Includes:

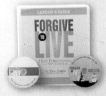

- Eight weeks of pre-designed PowerPoint™ presentations.
- Professionally designed customizable marketing materials and group handouts on CD-Rom.
- Training directly from author of *Forgive to Live* Dr. Dick Tibbits across six audio CDs.
- Media coverage DVD.
- CD-Rom containing all files in digital format for easy home or professional printing.
- A copy of the first study of its kind conducted by Stanford University and Florida Hospital showing a link between decreased blood pressure and forgiveness.

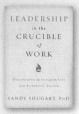

Leadership in the Crucible of Work (Hardcover)

What is the first and most important work of a leader? (The answer may surprise you.) In *Leadership in the Crucible of Work*, noted speaker, poet, and college president Dr. Sandy Shugart takes readers on an unforgettable journey to the heart of what it means to become an authentic leader.

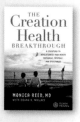

CREATION Health Breakthrough (Hardcover)

Blending science and lifestyle recommendations, Monica Reed, MD, prescribes eight essentials that will help reverse harmful health habits and prevent disease. Discover how intentional choices, rest, environment, activity, trust, relationships, outlook, and nutrition can put a person on the road to wellness. Features a three-day total body rejuvenation therapy and four-phase life transformation plan.

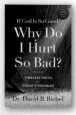

If God Is So Good, Why Do I Hurt So Bad? (Softcover)

In this powerful book, Dr. David Biebel leaves behind the all-too-familiar platitudes and instead offers the unvarnished truth about the pain of illness, death, divorce, financial ruin, and more. With keen insight and a compassionate outlook, Dr. Biebel puts God right by your side to help you see that your capacity for pain is an indicator of your potential for joy.

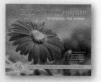

CREATION Health Devotional for Women (English)

Written for women by women, the *CREATION Health Devotional for Women* is based on the principles of whole-person wellness represented in CREATION Health. Spirits will be lifted and lives rejuvenated by the message of each unique chapter. This book is ideal for women's prayer groups, to give as a gift, or just to buy for your own edification and encouragement.

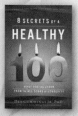

8 Secrets of a Healthy 100 (Softcover)

Can you imagine living to a Healthy 100 years of age? Dr. Des Cummings Jr., explores the principles practiced by the All-stars of Longevity to live longer and more abundantly. Take a journey through the 8 Secrets and you will be inspired to imagine living to a Healthy 100.